Understanding Managed Care

Understanding Managed Care

An Introduction for Health Care Professionals

Annette U. Rickel, Washington, D.C.
Thomas N. Wise, Falls Church, V.A.

8 figures in color, 2000

KARGER

Basel · Freiburg · Paris · London · New York ·
New Delhi · Bangkok · Singapore · Tokyo · Sydney

Annette U. Rickel, PhD

Clinical Professor of Psychiatry
Georgetown University Medical Center, Department of Psychiatry
3800 Reservoir Rd. NW 302A Kober Cogan, Washington, DC 20007, USA

Thomas N. Wise, MD

Medical Director, Behavioral Health Services
Chairman, Department of Psychiatry, Fairfax Hospital
Professor and Vice Chair,
Department of Psychiatry, Georgetown University School of Medicine
INOVA Health System, 3300 Gallows Road, Falls Church, VA 22046, USA

Library of Congress Cataloging-in-Publication Data
Rickel, Annette U., 1941–
Understanding managed care: an introduction for health care professionals / Annette U. Rickel,
Thomas N. Wise.
p.;cm.
Includes bibliographical references and index.
ISBN 3–8055–6960–2
1. Managed care plans (Medical care)   I. Wise, Thomas N.   II. Title.
[DNLM: 1. Managed Care Programs––United States.   W 130 AA1 R539u 1999]
RA413.R524   1999
362.1′04258––dc21

                                                             99-042843

      Bibliographic Indices. This publication is listed in bibliographic services, including Current Contents®
and Index Medicus.

      Drug Dosage. The authors and the publisher have exerted every effort to ensure that drug selection and
dosage set forth in this text are in accord with current recommendations and practice at the time of publication. However, in view of ongoing research, changes in government regulations, and the constant flow of
information relating to drug therapy and drug reactions, the reader is urged to check the package insert for
each drug for any change in indications and dosage and for added warnings and precautions. This is particularly important when the recommended agent is a new and/or infrequently employed drug.

      © Copyright 2000 by S. Karger AG, P.O. Box, CH–4009 Basel (Switzerland)
      Printed in Switzerland on acid-free paper by Reinhardt Druck, Basel
      ISBN 3–8055–6960–2

Table of Contents

Introduction

This book grew out of our teaching experiences with physicians and allied health care professionals who are graduating with in-depth knowledge of disease states and therapeutics, but little, if any practical knowledge of managed care systems. Managed care is so prevalent that in 1998, 85% of the U.S. working population was in some form of managed care network. Approximately 200,000 physicians are currently enrolled in managed care panels, which represents almost one third of the physicians in practice.

Despite such widespread participation, there has been a significant negative reaction by practitioners who see their autonomy and financial viability threatened. This has led the once conservative American Medical Association to endorse physician's unions to collectively bargain with managed care companies. This decision underscores the discontent that many of the 700,000 physicians in the U.S. have over the direction of the nation's health care system. Such discontent reflects the antagonism between health care professionals and the insurance industry, who paradoxically have been responsible for the economic forces leading to the technological growth of modern medicine.

How much do our students in health care, whether medical students, nurses in training, physical therapists or mental health professionals understand about managed care? Managed care is a broad generic term that encompasses many methods of managing both medical practice and cost. Perhaps there would be less discontent if health care professionals received training during their medical education about the current systems of managed care and methods of providing care within this new milieu.

A recent Medline search including the years 1990–97 yielded few citations concerning the teaching of the principles of managed care to students in medicine or the allied health care professions. When these students graduate, the managed care environment confronts them with an unknown language, a novel management structure, and an expanding scope of rules and regulations. Finding a job in a desirable location is increasingly difficult, and these new health care professionals are increasingly evaluated on their ability to understand the managed care environment.

This book is designed to serve either as a resource for teaching students or for independent and self-paced study. The initial chapters provide an overview of the changes in health care delivery in the United States, including the forces that are shaping the current environment. The basic structure and components of managed care organizations are then presented as well as the role of managing the health of these organization's populations. In addition, future challenges such as evidence-based medicine, medical ethics and quality measurement are also discussed. A series of cases based on a fictional family selecting a health plan and using its resources are provided to stress important topics; and a glossary section defines basic concepts frequently encountered in the managed care field. Key concepts significant to managed care are emboldened throughout the text and can be found clearly defined in the glossary. Key words are noted in the margins and important information highlighted in the text.

The authors would like to express their appreciation to the W.K. Kellogg Foundation for their support of this project, and to Robert DeVries, our Program Officer for his thoughtful perspective. Geoffry Gabriel's assistance on earlier versions of this manuscript was invaluable and the later work of Evvie Becker and Jody Evans aided in bringing our volume to completion.

We also are grateful for the generous support of the John D. and Catherine T. MacArthur Foundation and particularly thank Robert Rose, Director of Mental Health Policy and Research and Elizabeth McCormack, Vice Chairman of the Board of the Foundation for their guidance.

The MacArthur Foundation awarded us an educational grant to hold a regional training conference on 'Managed Care for New Health Professionals'. This book was used as the basis for the conference and provided an opportunity for us to determine its effectiveness. Presentations were made by Suzanne Gelber, Douglas Kay, Jeanne Matthews and John Wisniewski whose help and encouragement we gratefully acknowledge. From pre to post test, participants gained significantly in their knowledge of managed care as well as developed more positive attitudes toward this system of health care delivery.

With a firm and solid foundation gained from the use of this book, medical students and students in the allied health care professions will be more knowledgeable and comfortable in their role in managed care environments. Furthermore, with increased comfort levels and knowledge, it is believed that satisfaction with managed care will increase and positively effect direct patient care.

Annette U. Rickel and Thomas N. Wise

1. Historical Perspectives Leading to the Development of Managed Care

Introduction

The delivery of health care in the United States is undergoing dynamic change and revolution. Drugs that were once experimental are now commonplace, and some are sold without the need for a prescription. Diagnosis gradually moved from the bedside and examination room of earlier times, to magnetic resonance imaging, and other highly sophisticated procedures of modern days. Therapeutics can now treat the failing heart, the obstructed lungs, the schizophrenic mind. What was once miraculous is now often mundane and common. Indeed, the last half-century is witness to vast realignments in most aspects of medical practice and delivery in the United States.

Location of health care delivery gradually moved from the hospital bed to outpatient and extended care settings such as mall clinics, birth centers, urgent care centers and diagnostic radiology clinics – with new and novel locations appearing daily. Ever increasing numbers of physicians are earning their living as employees of health delivery corporations. At one time, it was sufficient for the health care professional to master the pathology and clinical therapeutics within their scope of practice. Now, they must be familiar with the concepts and vocabulary of managed care delivery.

For approximately the last 25 years, health care reform in the United States has become a major political, societal, ethical, economic and philosophical concern. As the 21st century approaches, it is difficult to find an area of professional or personal life that is not either touched or invaded by health care reform. As a nation, we are spending more dollars on health care per year, but getting less in return as the number of uninsured in the population increases by the hour, the day and the year (Blendon and Hyams, 1992). With spiraling costs came an inconsistent quality of care and the erosion of access to health care for a large segment of the population. As a result, managed care was introduced into traditional health indemnity plans in the 1970s as a means of controlling the rising health care costs. **Managed care**, a system of health care delivery that attempts to manage the cost, quality and access to health care, is now widely accepted as the norm while indemnity plans are rapidly being fazed out.

managed care

The popular press carries daily discussions on the threats, promises and provisions of this new, struggling delivery system for the nation's health. Unfortunately, the press tends to emphasize the dramatically bad outcomes of managed care, which in turn raises the public's wrath. It is the rare newspaper article that reflects an individual's satisfaction with his or her health care plan. Indeed, the medical journals, once a haven for basic and clinical scientific research, thought and discussion, are now filled with editorials and articles examining the managed care reform movement in a manner once reserved for mysterious new disease entities. The professional press contributes technical manuals designed to lead the practicing health care professional through the ever-increasing maze of regulations and vocabulary. Although there are many seminars to guide practicing clinicians through these turbulent times, there is minimal education about managed care for students in health care professions.

Finocchio et al. (1995) examined the attitudes of 300 physicians toward 16 areas of competency identified by the Pew Health Professions Commission as vital for practitioners 'to meet society's evolving health care needs'. More than 40 percent felt inadequately prepared to practice in a managed care environment when considering their undergraduate medical training. The authors concluded graduating physicians are 'likely to struggle with the demands placed on them by the emerging system, and without significant far-reaching reforms in medical education, students graduating in the future may feel less prepared to cope with their practice realities'. In addition, Veloski et al. (1996) reported that physicians in training or recently out of residency feel their educational experiences are not preparing them for a 'practice environment increasingly dominated by managed care'.

This chapter discusses historical perspectives necessary to understand the development of managed health care systems. These historical perspectives are examined as they relate to the cost, access and quality issues central to managed care. First, this chapter looks at the history of medical education and practice in the United States during the last 100 years with an emphasis on societal and economic pressures and constraints. With that background, the chapter then reviews the changes in the American hospital system, the origins of health insurance and the financing of **Medicare** and **Medicaid**.

History of Medical Education

The 19th century witnessed the rise of scientific medicine based on the scientific method so vital to a firm foundation for the clinical sciences. Virchow, the greatest pathologist of his time and clearly the dominant figure in European medicine during the later 1800s, integrated the clinical findings with experimental studies and brought scientific principles to bear on medical practice. Medical education in the United States in the early 1800s rested with a handful of medical schools, causing most physicians to learn their trade as apprentices to established physicians or to train in Europe (Raffel and Raffel, 1994). Physicians in the United States relied heavily on European colleagues for innovations in therapeutics and diagnostic techniques. As interest in medical training increased, so did the number of medical schools – most of them proprietary. The academic year was short, typically less than six months. Almost all students who applied were accepted, provided they could pay the tuition.

With the establishment of the Johns Hopkins University School of Medicine in 1893, a new instructional format was introduced. Hopkins required applicants to have a college degree, lengthened the instructional time to four years and integrated lectures with bedside teaching by full-time faculty members. No longer were lectures sufficient to teach medicine. Hopkins required its students to spend a sizable portion of their education in laboratory instruction to learn the scientific method and then train clinically in a carefully supervised hospital setting. The tradition of teaching at the bedside, rather than in an ambulatory setting' remains intact today (Bordley and Harvey, 1976).

While the Hopkins format spread to various medical schools across the country, in 1910 the Flexner Report entitled: *Medical Education in the United States and Canada,* critically examined 148 medical schools in the United States (Flexner, 1972). Flexner's conclusions were harsh and reported that the majority of medical schools produced poorly trained physicians. The report urged the closing of

_{scientific method}

_{Flexner Report}

many schools and the merging of the stronger ones with universities. Finally, it recommended that all medical schools should have an association with a hospital for clinical instruction of its students. In many ways the Flexner Report validated the innovations begun at Hopkins.

In the ten years after the publication of the Flexner report, the number of medical schools decreased from 131 to 85 (U.S. Department of Commerce, 1976). By 1940, there were approximately 135 physicians per 100,000 population whereas there were 160 per 100,000 in 1900. The reduction in physicians was most likely due to the decrease in the number of medical schools.

With the United States' entry into World War II, the number of medical schools remained constant at 80. Also, the number of physicians remained stable at an average of 135 per 100,000 population (U.S. Department of Commerce, 1976). During the war years, some medical schools had accelerated programs designed to grant degrees in three years instead of the traditional four. In addition, various medical schools developed, organized, and staffed general hospitals deployed during the war. With the increasing number of wounded soldiers, many of whom were paralyzed, missing limbs and blind, the need for rehabilitative medicine greatly increased. Advancements in physics during the war brought new and innovative diagnostic and therapeutic techniques to the realm of radiology, and led to significant strides in battlefield medicine. Overall, the war years were a productive time for American health care.

Health Professions
Education Assistance
Act

Comprehensive
Health Manpower
Training Act

Partially in response to the increasing portions of the United States underserved by health care providers, Congress passed the Health Professions Education Assistance Act in 1963 (Cooper, 1994). This legislation provided medical schools with money for construction and loans to students. Additional legislation in the form of the Comprehensive Health Manpower Training Act of 1971 gave further funds for building projects, scholarships, institutional aid, and the development of special instructional programs. This legislation benefited not only schools of medicine, but also schools of pharmacy, podiatry, dentistry, veterinary medicine, and osteopathy. Support funds related to the number of students enrolled increased and became available to all schools. In addition, government research grants also began to increase in 1971 – an important source of financing for most institutions.

By 1980, the number of allopathic schools had increased to 126 and the number of osteopathic schools to 14. In 1980, these schools graduated a total of 16,194 physicians. This represents an increase of 115% over the number of graduates in 1960. Furthermore, the number of active physicians per 100,000 population was 197 in 1980 – a 30 year high (Health, United States, 1996–97).

Changes in the American Hospital

While medical education underwent major upheavals, the concept of the hospital also changed. In the mid 1800s, fewer than 300 hospitals existed in the United States. Located mostly in large cities, a significant number of hospitals concentrated solely on the care of the mentally ill. Usually, the hospitals provided care on large wards, often unclean and understaffed. Since the hospital of that time had little to offer that could not be provided at home, those who could afford private medical care chose to be attended by their physicians at home. In many cases, the American hospital was a place to isolate those with infectious diseases, especially tuberculosis, and in large cities, this was typically a poor population. Thus, the American hospital of the late 1800s was still a place to be avoided.

Developments in technology changed the role the hospital played in health care delivery. With the widening knowledge base provided by the basic sciences came advancements in the clinical sciences. During a large percentage of the century, wound infection contributed largely to the morbidity and mortality associated with the practice of surgery. Many hospitals would not permit any operations that tended to have high rates of post-operative infections and deaths, especially abdominal procedures. It was not uncommon to have entire hospital surgical wards closed due to outbreaks of infection. As antiseptic surgery gradually gained acceptance, no longer was the risk of death from the surgical procedure greater than the risk of death from the disease process itself. Surgery moved from the kitchen table to the aseptic operating theater.

technology in medical practice

antiseptic surgery

The increased emphasis on technology in medical practice allowed for the systematization of diagnosis. To aid the physician in the diagnosis of many disease entities, both the electrocardiogram and the X-ray developed. In addition, the employment of technology helped to promote the increase in medical specialization so prevalent today.

systematization of diagnosis

The hospital of the early 20th century was also the scene of the development of the diagnostic laboratory, including services such as bacteriology, cellular pathology, and clinical chemistry. New technology enabled quicker and more accurate diagnosis, which in many cases speeded recovery time and decreased morbidity and mortality. By 1909, there were 4,359 hospitals in the United States with a total of 421,065 beds (Historical Statistics of the United States, 1976). This represented 4.7 beds per 1,000 population. No longer were these institutions seen as places housing the poor and the dying, no longer was a hospitalization a death sentence, and no longer were hospitals avoided by the middle and upper classes.

As outcomes improved, the hospital became the location of choice for the treatment of serious and life-threatening diseases. In addition, with the ongoing changes in medical education, many hospitals (especially those associated with a university-based medical school) became influential centers attracting well-known specialists of the day. With increased specialization, came hospitals and clinics devoted entirely to the diagnosis and treatment of certain disorders. The majority of these hospitals provided specialized nursing care not available in the general hospitals.

It is noteworthy that at the turn of the 20th century, charitable groups, especially religious orders, often managed the hospitals devoted largely to the treatment of the poor and indigent. These hospitals relied heavily upon generous support not only from various denominations, but also from the community and wealthy patrons (many of who would never consider obtaining treatment in the hospitals they supported!). The restrictions on hospital staff appointments led many physicians, especially surgeons, to develop proprietary hospitals designed only for the paying patient.

The concept of the for-profit hospital expanded as the middle and upper classes paid for services and treatment they now sought within a hospital setting. The decade between 1910 and 1920 saw an increase of 1,793 hospitals with an approximate doubling of the number of beds (Historical Statistics of the United States, 1976). Of these hospitals, 65% were general hospitals, 8% were mental hospitals, 1% were tuberculosis hospitals, and the remainder classified as 'other' (Historical Statistics of the United States, 1976).

Another significant factor that aided the overall improvement in American hospitals was the establishment of a hospital review system by the American College of Surgeons in 1918 (Bordley and Harvey, 1976). The College reviewed hospitals (usually having more than 100 beds) in a community and annually published a list for the

diagnostic laboratory

hospital review system

general public indicating which hospitals had met the stringent standards. The review included employing criteria for record keeping, activities of the medical staff, physical plants (including laboratories), surgical and anatomical pathology reviews, and therapeutic facilities. This was clearly the beginning of a widespread, systematized, and critical **peer review** of the nation's hospitals.

peer review

The relationship between the physician and patient also changed during this period. The yearly physical examination became the norm, especially after the First World War. It was now felt that this yearly visit to the physician could possibly detect underlying health problems before they became serious and possibly irreversible. This served to begin the establishment of a long term relationship between the physician and patient (Charap, 1981).

The Great Depression of the 1930s caused upheaval in all aspects of American life, including health care delivery. With high unemployment and the threat of financial ruin, the majority of American families could no longer afford medical care, especially hospital based services. People now depended on charity care. This signaled economic disaster for the proprietary hospitals, which had come to rely on patient generated revenues.

During the depression years, many hospitals closed their doors. The actual number of hospitals decreased in the years between 1929 and 1940, but the number of beds increased, reaching a high of 9.3 per 1,000 population in 1940 (U.S. Department of Commerce, 1976). Thus, the number of general hospital beds per 1,000 population remained fairly constant during this time period. However, the number of beds devoted to psychiatric patients increased by almost 50%.

The period after World War II saw a shortage of both hospitals and physicians. Construction of most new hospitals during the war years halted, as the war effort marshaled all needed resources. Physician shortage became especially acute in rural areas of the nation and sadly, continues today. In addition, the number of general practitioners decreased gradually because of retirement and the failure of medical graduates to enter primary care fields. Increasingly, young physicians selected specialization over general practice, urban areas over rural practice settings.

Enacted in 1946, the Hill–Burton Act provided federal subsidies under the Public Health Service Act to state governments for the construction of new hospitals and clinics and the modernization of existing structures. Under a complicated formula, the poorest states with the largest deficiencies in the number of hospitals and clinics received the greatest proportion of the federal funds. This Act re-

Hill-Burton Act

quired all applicants, private and local, to match each federal dollar with two dollars (Bordley and Harvey, 1976). In return, the institutions that benefited provided charity care in the amount equal to a predetermined percentage of their operating budgets.

In the period from its enactment to 1966, the Hill–Burton Act benefited approximately 4,700 various projects across the nation. With this landmark legislation, the federal government's focus shifted from providing funds for only military and veterans' hospitals to providing funds for all types of medical institutions (Henig, 1997).

In the twenty years from 1973 to 1993, the American hospital underwent numerous changes. The most significant change was the decrease in the number of hospitals, from 7,061 in 1972 to 6,467 in 1993. The bed rate per 1,000 population also decreased by 38%, with an average of 179 beds per hospital. The hospital segment hardest hit in terms of closures was the hospital with 24 beds or fewer, with a 50% decline in their numbers between 1971 and 1993. Occupancy rates dropped on the average by 13% for all hospitals and by 26% for profit hospitals. Federal hospitals only experienced a 4% decrease in occupancy during this same period. Expenses for hospitals, which exclude new construction, increased from $32.7 billion in 1972 to $301.5 billion in 1993 (Statistical Abstract of the United States, 1996). Finally, during this time period the number of personnel per 100 patients more than doubled.

How medical resources are utilized in the United States changed dramatically, not only in the last half century, but especially within the last twenty years. The nation's hospitals, private, public, and military, are undergoing major realignments under the strain of health care delivery. Surgical procedures once only done on an inpatient basis are now routinely performed as same-day surgeries in outpatient clinics. Between 1980 and 1993, the number of outpatient surgical operations performed in the setting of a short-stay hospital (typically less than 24 hours post op) more than tripled to approximately 55%. Where patients received their health care also changed. In 1993, some type of home health agency served approximately 1.5 million individuals, of whom most were 65 years of age and over, in their principal residence (Health, United States, 1996–97).

A major influence on the shaping of the American hospital in recent years is geographical location. Traditionally, major academic

academic health centers

health centers are in urban areas. Associated with schools of the health sciences, these centers are well funded and have sizable research programs in both the basic and clinical sciences and advanced technology and patient care. Such centers flourished under the reimbursement system that was in use 20 to 30 years ago. The system, in a crude sense, allowed almost unlimited use of medical resources and services. In addition to providing the resources and services, the academic health center also provided expensive specialty and subspecialty care. Iglehart (1993) reported a 1991 study estimating the average cost of care per patient per admission to an academic health center to be approximately $1,600 more than a similar admission to a non-teaching hospital. It is clear that to remain viable in the era of managed care reform and cost management, the academic health center should refocus its culture as a specialized service industry. This will pose especially difficult questions concerning the roles of research and clinical education. In the meantime, the community hospital is a viable alternative to the academic health center because of its lower average costs of care per patient.

By far, community hospitals outnumber academic health centers. In 1993, there were 5,261 community hospitals, representing 81% of the total hospitals in the United States. Of these, 60% were non-profit, 14% for profit and 26% owned and managed by state and local governments. A community hospital is by definition a non-Federal medical treatment center that can be a general hospital or a specialized treatment center. In addition, a community hospital provides its services to the public usually within a defined catchment area (Iglehart, 1993). Occupancy rates and the number of beds per 1,000 population steadily declined within the last twenty years for these hospitals. At the same time, expenses (excluding construction) increased by approximately 90%, and the number of employees rose by 80%. Not surprisingly, in the years between 1980 and 1993, 569 community hospitals closed their doors. This represented 96% of all hospital closures during the period.

community hospitals

While the statistics appear grim for the community hospital, the number of closures per year actually declined from 1988 to 1993. This decrease is most likely due to several factors. It probably indicates that those institutions that survived the late 1980s and early 1990s positioned themselves financially to meet the demands of the current health care delivery system. In particular, the number of outpatient visits, especially same-day surgeries, dramatically increased. This helped to offset revenue lost due to shorter hospital stays and decreases in third party reimbursements. However, the trend also contributed in part to the increase in the number of full-time employees. In addition, some institutions converted previous short-stay beds into long-care chronic beds, noting the increase in nursing home beds.

Origins of Health Insurance

Health insurance originated in 1929 in Baylor, Texas with the establishment of the forerunner of the Blue Cross Insurance Company. Schoolteachers in Baylor enrolled in the first group health insurance plan which provided a set number of days of hospitalization for a set yearly fee.

employer paid health
insurance

As the nation industrialized for the war effort, employers and their representatives began to include health insurance as a provision in benefit packages. By 1943, approximately 19% of the civilian population had protection under hospitalization insurance. From this a trend began toward employer paid health insurance premiums – a practice which continues to this day.

While those who were employed or could afford the out-of-pocket expense fared well with the rise in medical coverage, the poor continued to fall mostly outside the insurance safety net. Since the early 1900s, medical care delivery for the poor and uninsured did not change drastically. This segment of the population still had the same choices that were available to an earlier generation – go without, or rely on charity care provided at large municipal institutions. Often these municipal institutions were understaffed, overworked, with resources stretched to the limit.

To cope with the costs of medical care, prepaid plans developed that were a form of insurance provided by the physicians. One example of an early system of managed care originated in Elk City, Oklahoma in 1929, where a rural cooperative of farmers formed a community organization to offer health care to the members at discounted rates. An annual dues schedule covered the costs of medical care. Similarly in 1929, two Los Angeles physicians entered into a prepaid contract to provide comprehensive health services to 2,000 employees of a water company.

Several other examples of prepaid group practice plans developed between 1930 and 1960 despite opposition from local medical societies. In 1937, the Group Health Association formed in Washington, D.C. and in 1942, the Kaiser-Permanente Medical Care Program formed to provide health care for the ship yard and, dock workers in Northern California and their dependents (Smillie, 1991). Other systems followed, such as the establishment in 1947 of the Health Insurance Plan of Greater New York and the Group Health Cooperative of Puget Sound in Seattle, Washington.

The passage of the HMO Act of 1973 laid the groundwork for increased control of medical care delivery by third party payers. This Act defined the characteristics of what a **Health Maintenance Organization** (HMO) should have, including an organized system for providing health care, an agreed set of fundamental and supplemental health maintenance and treatment services and a voluntary group of participants. The Act virtually encouraged group formation, cost containment activities and concern for the quality of health care being delivered in these systems. At the same time, the HMO Act enabled managed care plans to expand enrollments through health care programs financed by loans, grants and contracts. Currently, managed care is so prevalent that there is now over 85% of the U.S. working population involved in some form of network (U.S. Department of Health and Human Services, 1997).

Health Maintenance Organization Act

Financing Medicare and Medicaid

In partial reaction to the growing disparity in health care benefits, the Johnson Administration and Congress created the Medicare and Medicaid programs in 1965. This action brought to a partial resolution a debate over federal sponsorship of health care financing that began during the administration of Franklin Roosevelt. Under these plans, health care became initially available to the elderly and the poor, two segments of the population hardest hit by the lack of coverage for medical expenses.

Medicare is the federal health insurance program for Americans over the age of 65. It is divided into two segments: a mandatory Part A which covers hospital costs, and an optional Part B designed to cover physicians fees and outpatient costs. Both the federal and state governments jointly administer Medicaid, a program for Americans

Medicare

Medicaid

in low-income brackets. With the development of these programs, the federal and state governments stepped in to the medical insurance maze. This forever changed the relationship between the government and the medical community!

The enactment of Medicare and Medicaid in 1965 further advanced the support of managed care by the federal government. Physician systems sprung up to provide the physicians with a means of delivering care and securing timely payment. With the founding of Medicare and Medicaid, the federal government began to finance a large portion of long-term care. Medicaid pays for approximately 47% of the total for all nursing home care and respectively 27% of home health care, while Medicare pays for approximately 5% of nursing home care and 45% of home health care (Weiner, 1994). Medicare expenditures for home health care are projected to reach $14.5 billion in 1996.

chronic illness

The question of long-term health care in the setting of managed care with Medicare remains unanswered. Current Medicare home health care regulations favor acute illness over **chronic illness**, refusing to pay for most services utilized to maintain the chronically ill at home. Medicare does not have an incentive to reimburse for continuing home health care, especially if the alternative is nursing home care. Once the chronically ill patient enters a nursing home, he will be forced to utilize private funds. With the private funds exhausted, the patient then becomes eligible for Medicaid. Thus, cost shifting between Medicare and Medicaid occurs, an attractive alternative for the managed care organization.

During its first full year of operation in 1966, Medicare had 19.1 million enrollees, 3.7 million (19%) of whom actually used the benefits under the newly created program. By comparison, in 1999 Medicare had 39 million enrollees (93% increase since 1966) with 30.1 million (82%) users. It is estimated that by the year 2030, the number of enrollees will be close to 70 million (U.S. Bureau of the Census, 1993). If the current utilization pattern holds stable, 57.4 million enrollees will be actual users in the year 2030. However, the expectation is that Medicare will be solvent only to the year 2005.

In 1994, Medicare had expenditures for personal health care of $166.1 billion, representing an increase of $17.1 billion from 1993. With 30.1 million users in 1994, this represents an average spending of $5.537 per user. However, the Health Care Financing Administration (HCFA) estimates that 11% of the enrollees (4.06 million) are responsible for 73% ($121.3 billion) of the payments. This averages to $26,359 per individual. There is also disparity between average payments for individuals in different age cohorts. In 1993, the average Medicare payment for an individual over 85 years of age was approximately 2.3 times greater than the average payment for an individual 65 to 66 years old (Health, United States, 1996–97). Medicare expenditures for hospital care, physician services, home health care, and other professional services all increased in 1994. Medicare was responsible for 30% of hospital revenue and 20% of physician payments in 1994.

Funding for Medicare is unique among Federal programs in that it does not rely only on appropriations from the general tax revenues. Instead, Medicare comprises a hospital insurance program (Part A) and a supplementary medical insurance program (Part B), each with its own trust fund. The hospital program covers home health care, hospice care, inpatient care, and outpatient skilled nursing care. The medical program covers physician fees and the majority of outpatient care. Employees and employers each contribute a 1.45% (for a total of 2.9% per employee) payroll tax to support the hospital trust fund. In 1994, this contribution accounted for 87.3% of the payments into the hospital trust fund. An additional 9.8% came from interest revenue. The medical fund receives its revenues through a monthly premium paid by each enrollee ($41.10 in 1994) and through general revenues. In 1994, the general revenue contributed to 65.1% of the medical fund resources while the payment of premiums generated 31.3%.

Medicare Part A
Medicare Part B

It is important to note that Medicare managed care enrollment has doubled since 1993, even though it began more than a decade ago. Almost 15% of the Medicare population is in a managed care plan, a staggering 5.6 million Medicare **beneficiaries**. Also, as of September 1997, the total number of Medicare managed care plans has quadrupled since 1991 (Health Care Financing Administration, 1995).

Medicare managed care

beneficiaries

In response to the significant increase of Medicare managed care enrollees, President Clinton signed legislation on August 5, 1997 that establishes new health care options entitled Medicare + Choice. The Balanced Budget Act of 1997 means more managed care plans are available, especially affecting the five states that currently do not offer Medicare managed care plans (Alaska, Maine, Mississippi, South Dakota and Wyoming). To address the need of increasing the

Medicare + Choice

prevalence of Medicare managed care plans in underserved and rural areas, the Act allows for more choices for Medicare patients, such as offering **Preferred Provider Organization Plans** (American Association of Retired Persons (AARP, 1997).

Preferred Provider
Organization Plans

The new legislation also affects the reimbursement payments to the managed care organizations. Reimbursements will increase to those areas with lower medical costs, while conversely, those cities with normally high reimbursement costs will decrease in an attempt to even out the reimbursement distribution across the country.

Another significant change that the Act introduces is the ability of patients to switch from Medicare managed care plans back to **fee-for-service** plans at the beginning of each month. The new legislation states that by 2002, patients can only change plans within a six month time frame per year, unless there is just cause. The following year, 2003, patients have a three month time frame in which to change plans per year. However, new Medicare enrollees will be allowed to switch from managed care plans to fee-for-service plans and purchase Medigap insurance within the first twelve months of signing up for Medicare. Yet, after a year, the patients can only change plans during a three month time frame (AARP, 1997).

fee-for-service

The Medicaid program provides services for both disabled and low-income individuals. In 1994, there were 35.1 million Medicaid recipients, of which approximately 17 million were children under age 21, 10 million were disabled, aged, and/or blind individuals, and 8 million were adults covered under the Aid to Families with Dependent Children (AFDC). Medicaid covered an additional 1.0 million individuals that did not belong to one of the above cohorts. The disabled, aged, and blind are eligible based on disability status, income, and/or medical expenses. It is interesting to note that while the majority of the Medicaid recipients were children and adults in families with dependent children, it was the disabled, aged, blind group that received the majority of program payments in 1994. Average payments in 1994 ranged from $152 for medical screening of children to $52,269 for services in an intermediate care facility for the mentally retarded (Health, United States, 1996–97). In the same year, approximately 25% of Medicaid payments went to nursing facilities, 25% to hospitals, and 7% to home health care.

The federal, state and local governments jointly fund the Medicaid program. The states receive matching funds from the federal government and must meet minimum requirements set forth by the Federal government. As states faced increasing expenditures for Medicaid programs, managed care became an attractive option (Hurley, Freund and Paul, 1993). In 1990 there were approximately 2.1 million Medicaid recipients enrolled in various managed care plans. By 1995, managed care plans covered 12 million recipients, representing approximately one third of all individuals enrolled in Medicaid (HCFA, 1995).

It is important to note that Medicaid managed care enrollment doubled between 1991 and 1994, even though it has been in effect since 1965. Because each state develops and coordinates its own Medicaid program within Federal mandates, there is a substantial increase in Medicaid managed care plans as states grapple with financing their Medicaid programs. For example, the state of Minnesota developed an innovative project entitled 'Minnesota Senior Health Options'. This five-year pilot program permits Minnesota to combine the purchase of both Medicaid and Medicare services in the same contract. Managed care plans are paid a capitated rate per individual to cover basic health care services for Medicaid or Medicare enrollees. The program has the potential to drastically alter the financing and delivery of health services on both the state and federal level, as Minnesota demands that the managed care organizations provide integrated care. As state and local governments continue to seek ways to navigate the costs of Medicaid, managed care will continue the inroads made during the early 1990s.

Medicaid managed care

Summary and Conclusions

This overview of the history of medical education and practice in the United States over the past 100 years, as well as the changes in the American hospital system, the financing of health insurance, and the enactment of Medicare and Medicaid, provides a background from which to examine the factors that contributed to the development of systems of managed care.

The 19th century saw the rise of scientific medicine while the 20th century ushered in the development of technology and the diagnostic laboratory. The Depression of the 1930s caused upheaval in health care delivery, as many Americans could not afford medical care which resulted in the closing of numerous hospitals. The Hill-Burton Act of 1946 addressed the shortage of physicians and hospitals after World War II and the creation of Medicare and Medicaid in 1965 brought health care financing to the state and federal level.

The chapter also reviews the growth of managed care from its beginnings in 1930 to the present. The financing of Medicare, which is expected to be solvent only to the year 2005, and the increasing expenditures for Medicaid programs were further discussed.

2. Why Managed Care?

The U.S. health care system during the past 15 years has undergone astounding changes that might be described as revolutionary. Physicians and hospitals lost their dominance and their authority was transferred to managed care organizations. This phenomenon came about because employers demanded that providers and insurers manage health care costs more effectively.

Prior to 1980, physicians and hospitals had carte blanche in providing a range of health care services and were able to charge what the market would bear for these services. As providers charges increased, health insurers increased the premiums to employers in order to recoup their losses. Health care costs did not become an issue at this time because of the strength of the economy between 1945 and 1973. Employers of union and non-union shops felt little pressure to contain insurance premium increases. However, health care expenditures beginning in the 1960s were skyrocketing at twice the rate of inflation. Prestigious publications such as the Harvard Business Review, Fortune, Business Week and the Wall Street Journal forewarned of the major problems of escalating health care costs.

Persistent health care inflation and a stammering economy forced health care costs in the 1980s to the top of the agenda in America's corporate board rooms. Steps were taken to shift a larger percentage of health care premiums to employees by increasing **deductibles** and **co-payments** in 'fee-for-service' plans. This became a major source of contention between employer and employees. Nevertheless, employers health care costs increased dramatically (e.g., 19% in 1988, and 17% in 1989 and 1990). As a percentage of total wages and salaries, health insurance expenditures rose to 9% from 2% in 1965. The spending of health services as a percentage of

deductibles
co-payments

the Gross Domestic Product was also staggering (see page 24 for a more in-depth discussion of the GDP).

These increased health care costs put American industry at a global competitive disadvantage, particularly the big three automakers in their battle for market share with Japan. For example, health insurance comprised $700 of the costs of an American car whereas the health insurance costs of a Japanese car amounted to only $200.

It was the bold step of Allied Signal, a corporation closely associated with the automotive industry, that provided the impetus to change corporate Americas attitude towards the absorption of increased health care costs. Allied transferred 80,000 employees and dependents into a managed care plan – Cigna's Health Maintenance Organization which saved the company millions of dollars.

Allied Signals significant action started the movement among corporate America to guide employees into managed care plans. By 1996, one hundred million American workers received their health care coverage through managed care plans. This acceleration of managed care seriously curtailed employers offering of 'fee-for-service' indemnity insurance plans. Therefore, one of the main reasons for the introduction of managed care in the U.S. work force was employers concern that health care costs were destroying profit margins.

This chapter will present demographic changes and disease pattern shifts in the population contributing to increased U.S. health care expenditure trends. The chapter also chronicles health care reform in the U.S. at the federal and state level that attempts to improve quality and access of health care and discusses how other industrialized nations provide citizens with cost effective health care.

Demographic Changes

Americans are living longer, and the numbers are impressive. The average life expectancy for a person born in 1990 is approximately 75 years. The percentage of the population over 65 is approaching 15%. It is estimated that by the year 2030, this group will account for 30% of the population (U.S. Senate Special Committee on Aging, 1991). As can be seen in fig. 2.1, by the year 2030 there will be approximately 70 million people over the age of 65, almost double the aged population in the year 2000.

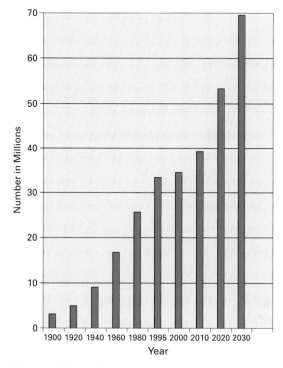

Fig. 2.1 Number of Persons 65 and Over

Source: U.S. Bureau of the Census: 'Sixty-Five Plus in America', P23–178 RV; 'Population Projections of the United States by Age, Sex, Race and Hispanic Origin: 1993 to 2050', P25–1104.

What do these numbers mean to the health care delivery system? Few dispute the fact that we are becoming an aged population. However, what appears most significant is that our elderly population is aging within itself (James, 1997). If estimates hold true, we can expect by the year 2000 that within the age 65+ population, the majority will be over the age of 75. This portion of the population is typically sicker, requiring more frequent hospitalizations for both acute and chronic diseases. In addition, an aging population experiences reductions in the activities of daily living (feeding, bathing, dressing, toileting, etc.) with increasing functional limitations. Figure 2.2 indicates that with advancing age the percentage of people needing assistance increases dramatically.

aging U.S. population

In 1993, the U.S. Center for Health Statistics reported that of the civilian non-institutionalized population over 65 years of age receiving home health care, 54.5% required help bathing, 47.1% needed assistance with dressing and 35.2% required help with transfer in/out of a bed or chair (Statistical Abstract of the United States, 1995).

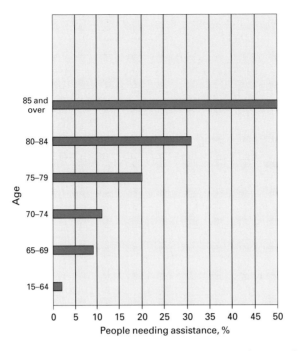

Fig. 2.2 Percentage of Persons Needing Assistance with Everyday Activi-
tes, By Age: 1990–1991 (Civilian Non-institutional Population)

Source: U.S. Census Bureau, Last Revision: May 13, 1997.

In 1998, persons 65 and over received approximately one-third of
the entire annual expenditure for health care in the United States (U.S.
Senate Special Select Committee on Aging, 1989). Since Medicare
covers the majority of the population over 65 years of age, (and as this
segment of the population will continue to increase), it is reasonable
to assume the annual expenditures for this group will increase. However, as Himmelstein and Woolhandler (1994) point out, the elderly
still spend a substantial percentage of their income, (approximately
18% in 1998), on health care beyond Medicare coverage. Thus, to only
examine Medicare as a gauge of the health care dollar spent on the
elderly of this nation misses a sizable out-of-pocket portion.

Disease Pattern Changes

Since the turn of the 20th century, the reasons Americans were
dying changed drastically. In 1900, infectious diseases were among the

leading causes of death in the United States, responsible for approximately 600 deaths per 100,000 population. The most significant were pneumonia and influenza (202.2 deaths per 100,000), followed by tuberculosis (194.4 deaths per 100,000), and intestinal infections (142.7 deaths per 100,000) (U.S. Department of Commerce, 1976). Major cardiovascular and renal diseases were also significant causes of death at the turn of the century, accounting for 345.2 deaths per 100,000.

Deaths from respiratory infections began a gradual decline until the influenza pandemic in 1918. During that year, there were almost triple the number of deaths due to pneumonia and influenza that had occurred in 1900. Both tuberculosis and intestinal infection deaths continued a slow decline from 1900 on, never again reaching the high numbers seen at the turn of the century. However, the number of deaths attributable to major cardiovascular and renal diseases continued to increase over the years. In addition, deaths due to various malignant neoplasms increased from 64.0 deaths per 100,000 population in 1900 to 162.8 deaths per 100,000 population in 1970. By 1970, deaths due to other infectious agents such as typhoid and paratyphoid, scarlet fever and streptococcal infections, diphtheria, whooping cough, and measles decreased to less than 0.05 deaths per 100,000 (U.S. Department of Commerce, 1976).

From 1970, the troubling death rate due to various malignancies continued to increase, reaching a high of 205.8 deaths per 100,000 population in 1993 (U.S. Department of Commerce, 1996). This represented 23.4% of all deaths by selected causes, second only to deaths due to major cardiovascular diseases (32.6%). Since 1970, malignancies of the respiratory and intrathoracic organs, chiefly lung carcinoma, attributed to the greatest increase in neoplastic related deaths.

cardiovascular and neoplastic related deaths

The death rate due to major cardiovascular diseases actually decreased from 496.0 deaths per 100,000 in 1970 to 366.3 deaths per 100,000 in 1993 (U.S. Department of Commerce, 1996). Also, deaths due to ischemic heart disease, cerebrovascular diseases, atherosclerosis, and rheumatic fever and rheumatic heart disease significantly decreased. However, deaths due to hypertension and hypertensive heart disease increased during this 23-year period.

The early 1980s saw the emergence of HIV disease and AIDS. Originally focused in the homosexual community, this disease now claims victims in all strata of the population – women, heterosexuals, bisexuals, children, infants, and the elderly with increasing numbers (Morbidity and Mortality Weekly Reports, 1996). As the number of HIV infected individuals rose in the 1980s, this increase fueled concern over the impact these individuals might have on the health care

HIV and AIDS

delivery system. Hardy et al. (1986) completed a study of the financial impact of the first 10,000 AIDS cases in the United States. They demonstrated that from the time of initial diagnosis to the time of death, the average cost of direct medical care was $147,000. This figure, in combination with the uncertain number of infected individuals and an uncertain disease progression, led to both lay and professional concerns over the cost of health care for the AIDS population.

Hellinger (1993) also examined the lifetime costs of treating an individual with AIDS and estimated the cost to be approximately $120,000. However, in the ten years since the publication of the above statistic, the initial concerns of doom never fully materialized. The direct medical cost is realistically between 2 and 3% of the national health care expenditure. Nevertheless, as an increasing number of AIDS patients lose or exhaust their private insurance and become dependent on Medicaid, how health care is supplied to these individuals will become an issue of financing, not so much of cost. In 1993, Medicaid paid for approximately 90% of the children with AIDS and approximately 40% of the adult AIDS cases (Washington Outlook, 1993).

It is virtually impossible to predict the full impact the AIDS epidemic will have on health care delivery in the next ten years. Because AIDS affects practically every organ system, there is not a single branch of medicine not called on to treat various complications of the disease. In addition, with the introduction of new therapeutics, the natural progression of the disease is changing. Also, procedures and therapeutics once performed only on an inpatient basis are now administered in clinic settings and at home. Thus, the need lessened considerably for inpatient beds. Finally, as the disease takes hold in various populations (such as the elderly and the homeless) with established disease patterns, new issues concerning treatment management arise. These treatment options include palliative care and hospice.

How care gets distributed among these competing disease states remains a question of our time, and answering that question is what managed care is forced to do every day.

U.S. Health Expenditures

During the last ten years, health care delivery underwent major revolutionary changes (Starr, 1992). How the U.S. pays for its health care and how much the U.S. pays are issues central to the movement for managed care reform. There were realignments in professional practices, reimbursement scales and methods, and institutional care (Goodman and Musgrave, 1992). Expenditures for health care in 1995 represented 13.6% of the gross domestic product (GDP). While this was the largest percentage of the GDP to date, it actually represented a slowing of the rate of annual increase to approximately 6.4%. In 1992, the increase was approximately 10% (Health, United States, 1996–97).

National health expenditures increased from $26.9 billion in 1960 to $988.5 billion in 1995 (see fig. 2.3). In 1960, $141 was spent per individual, while the 1995 figure represents an average of $3,621 spent per individual. While these increased numbers are dramatic, it is instructive to examine the increase in federal payments for health care as a percentage of total government expenditures.

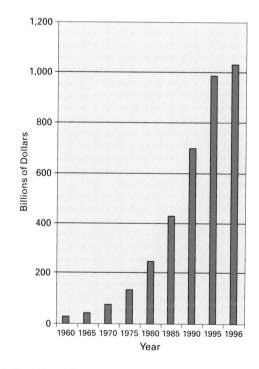

Fig. 2.3 National Health Care Expenditures

Source: Health, United States 1996–1997. National Center for Health Statistics.

In 1960, health expenditures amounted to 3.3% of total federal out-lays. By 1966 with Medicare and Medicaid in full operation, the per-centage increased to 5.4% with an expenditure of $219 per individual.

During the Bicentennial year of 1976, the percentage reached the double digits for the first time – 10.7%. By 1995, the Federal govern-ment spent 20% of its total expenditures on health care delivery – an all time high (Health, United States, 1996–97). When examined by decades, these trends indicate that the 1960s saw the steepest increa-se – approximately 155%. This increase is understandable, as the Federal government became the largest third party payer for health care beginning in the 1960s. During the 1970s, the overall increase declined to a total of 36%, and during the 1980s it declined to 26%. Even with the emphasis on cost management and containment, the first four years of the 1990s saw the sharpest increase (27%) in thir-ty years. Despite these percentages, 37 million Americans have no health insurance and an additional 50 million are underinsured.

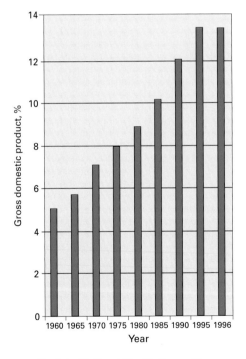

Fig. 2.4 National Health Expenditures as a Percentage of the GDP.
Source: Health, United States 1996–97. National Center for Health Statistics.

Gross Domestic Product. By definition, the GDP is the value of all final goods and services produced in the economy during a given period of time (quarter or year) and are a measure of economic activity. Typically, health expenditures as a percentage of the GDP measure the impact of health care spending on the nation's economy. As in fig. 2.4, in 1960 health expenditures represented 5.1% of the GDP and by 1995, this percentage rose to 13.7. This represents an average increase of 2.5% per year. Between 1990 and 1994, there was an average yearly increase of 4.0%. However, between 1993 and 1994, the percentage only increased by 0.1%, a trend not experienced since 1983. This was most likely due to a substantial increase in the GDP ($380.8 billion) and the lowest increase in national health care expenditures in seven years (Statistical Abstract of the United States, 1996). Of all industrial nations, the United States remains the leader in percentage of GDP devoted to health care expenditures.

Hospital Services. These were the largest component of health care expenditures in 1995 – $338.5 billion dollars, that was 36% of the total expenditures, a 4.4% increase over expenditures in 1993. In the four-year period from 1990 to 1994, hospital expenditures increased by 32%, with an average increase of 8.0% per year. Between 1960 and 1990, costs increased from 9.3 billion to 256.4 billion. The sharpest 10-year increase occurred in the decade between 1970 and 1980, with an average increase of 27% per year. In 1960, 20.7% ($1.9 billion) of hospital care expenditures were paid out of pocket, and 79.3% ($7.4 billion) were paid by third parties, including Federal, State, and local payments. By 1994, out of pocket payments dropped to 2.9% ($9.8 billion) and third party payments increased to 97.1%.

While hospital expenditures continue to increase overall, the 4.4% increase between 1993 and 1994 actually represented a four-year low. Clearly, the deceleration is due to many factors. Hospital revenue from inpatient stays decreased by 1.0% in 1994. For all ages, the average length of the inpatient stay decreased from 6.2 days in 1993 to 6.0 days in 1994. In addition, the admissions per 1,000 population remained stable at 122 for the years between 1992 and 1994. When this data is divided into two separate age groups, those above 65 years and those below 65, two separate trends become evident. While the average length of stay for the over 65 age group continues to decrease, the actual number of admissions increased by an average of 2.2 % per year. This is in contrast to the under age 65 segment, which, for the first time in 10 years recorded an increase in hospital admissions in 1994.

Outpatient Procedures. In stark contrast to inpatient revenues, outpatient revenues continued in a steady yearly increase since 1985. This trend will most likely continue as the number of outpatient procedures, especially surgical procedures, increases (Gold, 1995). Historically, HMOs had lower hospital admission rates than indemnity plans. With increased enrollment in HMOs, it is expected that inpatient revenues will continue to decelerate over time (Miller and Luft, 1994). However, as indemnity plans continue to adopt certain procedures utilized by HMOs in controlling hospital costs, especially pre-certification, it is likely that these two types of coverage will become indistinguishable in terms of outpatient hospitalization rates (Dellinger, 1992). This will probably contribute to a second wave of decreased inpatient revenue as the indemnity plans fully adopt these measures.

Long-term Care. With an increasing portion of the population over age 65, concerns over the financing of long-term care (nursing

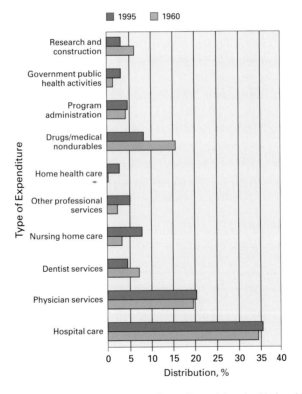

Fig. 2.5 Type of Expenditure Comprising the National Health Expenditures
Source: Health, United States 1996–97. National Center for Health Statistics.

homes and home health care) become paramount when discussing managed care reform. Figure 2.5 points out that the percentage of this type of care, as part of the National Health Expenditures, tripled since 1960. Within this portion of the population is a large cohort of elderly individuals with limitations due to chronic diseases. Most often these limitations involve a substantial amount of morbidity associated with loss of mobility, a loss of both involuntary and voluntary muscle control, and impairment in cognitive functions.

Of the two main types of long-term care, Americans utilize the nursing home more than home health care. There are currently more than 33,000 nursing homes in the United States, the majority under proprietary control. In 1991, these facilities had an average of 58 beds with 90% occupancy. The South has the highest number of homes, followed by the Midwest, West, and Northeast regions. Hospital-based nursing homes numbered 767 in 1991 with 51,897 residents (Statistical Abstract of the United States, 1996).

nursing home vs. home health care

Expenditures for home health care drastically grew, totaling $30.932 billion in 1994, and accounting for 3.2% of total health expenditures. This figure represents a 107% increase over expenditures in 1990, an average increase of 27% per year. Of the total home health expenditures in 1994, 85% was non-hospital based (freestanding public or private agencies). Of the total spent, Medicare paid 42% and Medicaid paid 16%. Since 1990, Medicare has increased its payments by approximately 57% per year. Currently, Medicare is the largest purchaser of home health care, approximately 3.5 million patients receive home health care benefits (Freudenheim, 1995). As the population continues to age, this number will most likely increase. In addition, as the range of services provided by home health agencies broadens, the access to at-home technology by the chronically ill will rise.

Comparison of Industrialized Nations Health Care Systems

Given these escalating medical costs, can the United States learn from other industrialized nations on how to provide citizens with cost effective health care coverage? As noted previously, the U.S. spends approximately 14% of the GDP on health care; whereas Germany, France, and Canada spend 8–9%, and Australia, Japan and Great Britain spend 6–8% respectively.

Yet, despite all that the United States spends on health care, it has the highest infant mortality rate and the lowest life expectancy rate within these industrialized nations (Bok, 1996). In comparing the United States with these other industrialized countries, the cost of medical care is clearly highest in the U.S. However, over 15% of the United States population is uninsured, and this rising percentage is significantly higher than that found in other industrialized nations (Bok, 1996). These factors led President Clinton in 1993 to undertake health care reform and to propose the Health Security Bill.

Clinton's Health
Security Bill

The Clinton Task Force for National Health Care Reform presented a proposal to overhaul the current system. Clinton's plan protected and expanded quality of care and included the following principles: 1. provide Americans with the security of knowing that they will have health coverage even if they switch jobs, lose their job or have a pre-existing condition; 2. allow consumers to choose a health plan from a variety of options; 3. hold doctors and hospitals accountable with a consumer **'report card'** for each health plan and eliminate fraud and abuse by imposing stiff criminal penalties on the profiteers; 4. implement malpractice reform to reduce the defensive medicine that drives up costs; and 5. simplify paperwork by creating a single insurance form.

report card

Clinton's Health Security Bill did not pass. Congress felt the proposal was too complex and big, with the establishment of an independent national health board to set a global budget for health care services at the federal level that would then be allocated to state and regional Health Alliances. Clinton's plan recommended financing of more than half of the health care reform proposal through savings in Medicaid and Medicare. Also, the plan suggested a cigarette tax to help pay for long-term care for the elderly and disabled, as well as asking employers and employees to take some responsibility for paying for health care. Again, the legislators had serious concerns about these ways to finance the proposal.

While a large-scale federal effort to reform health care in the United States did not occur, some strides did on a smaller scale. For example, the Health Insurance Portability and Accountability Act of 1996 passed thanks to the efforts of Senators Kennedy and Kassenbaum. Effective July 1, 1997, the key aspects of this Act assured that Americans could carry health insurance from job to job and are covered for pre-existing conditions when switching health plans. Another significant federal effort in health care reform is the Mental Health Parity Act of 1996 that Senators Domenici and Wellstone moved forward. The Act, effective January 1, 1998, prevents health

Health Insurance
Portability and
Accountability Act

Mental Health
Parity Act

plans from placing an unequal dollar limit on mental health services vs. medical/surgical treatment on an annual or lifetime basis. This legislation does not effect inpatient or outpatient visit limits and does not apply to substance abuse or chemical dependency treatment.

Legislative debate on how to accomplish health care reform continues on a Federal level. This debate centers on whether access to quality health care should focus on individuals based on income (e.g., the working poor) or by age (e.g., the elderly). As illustrated by the large number of proposals in Congress to expand health insurance to children, including President Clinton's 'Kiddiecare', it is evident that children are the priority.

Also, states are proposing innovative health care reforms, particularly those aimed at uninsured children and families. For example, the state of Arkansas proposed 'Kids First', a preventive health benefit package aimed at children in poverty. Florida is trying to expand their state subsidized health insurance program entitled 'Healthy Kids Corporation', which makes low cost insurance available through school systems. In addition, South Carolina introduced a bill that would require the state to cover the cost of emergency services for children (American Political Network, 1997)

Kentucky, Minnesota, Connecticut and Colorado enacted significant health care reform legislation but must overcome major hurdles posed by the Employee Retirement Income Security Act (ERISA) of 1974 before enacting their laws. However, Florida, New York, Tennessee, Texas and Oregon are all implementing health care reform legislation passed since 1989. For example, the state of Oregon set the **benchmark** for universal coverage by extending health services to a large number of residents. Under Oregon's coverage, more individuals are in Medicaid managed care plans with a prioritized list of the medical conditions that will be covered. Only 565 of the 696 medical conditions normally covered by Medicaid are paid for by the State (Bodenheimer, 1997).

Among the industrialized nations, the United States is the only country that relies on both the private markets and the public sectors to determine the type, quality and amount of medical care provided. Other nations allow governments to intervene and play a lead role in determining the cost and type of medical care. Taxes fund the medical costs, and all citizens, regardless of whether or not they are in the work force, are eligible for health care. However, each country developed a different way to control costs.

One of the oldest health care systems in Europe is Germany's universal coverage system that has, as a major component, the 'sick-

benchmark

Germany's universal coverage system

ness funds'. Regulated by the government, these funds are comparable to U.S. health insurance firms and are not-for-profit organizations. Ninety percent of the German population are members of these funds, as it is compulsory unless one's salary is high enough to opt for private insurance. Payroll taxes on employers and employees, as well as retired individuals' pensions in an aggregate amount agreed to by the National Council, finance the system. Each 'sickness fund' must negotiate fee schedules with medical providers and hospitals.

The German government is continually initiating cost control measures, but implementation of these measures rested with the sickness funds and the physician associations. In the mid 1980s, cost measures included capitation for physician reimbursement, however, many experts feel this did not reduce the delivery of medical services. Furthermore, during these same years hospital construction was cut back while hospital beds remained constant. To keep pharmaceutical costs down, patients receive the lowest-priced generic drug or otherwise they must pay the cost difference if they want a non-generic drug (Huefner and Battin, 1992).

France's universal health care delivery system

The French universal health care delivery system, similar to the German system, is set up to reward workers and is financed by them. However, in the past sixty years coverage expanded to benefit the self-employed, the unemployed and the retired. Insurance funds established by the state reimburse health care providers on a fee-for-service basis. Negotiations between physicians' associations and the French government determine fee schedules. Although this structure allows physicians a good deal of autonomy, behind these insurance funds are the National Ministries of Health, Finance and Social Security that make significant budgetary decisions.

During the 1980s, mounting health care costs also became a primary concern for the French government. To constrain costs, the French restricted the number of medical school graduates. This measure assumed that medical use would soon be limited if the supply of physicians was limited. Other cost containment measures initiated include: global budgets for hospitals, constraining the income of health care providers, and assessing user fees to financially-able patients for each day they spent in the hospital (Huefner and Battin, 1992).

United Kingdom's National Health Service

The United Kingdom's National Health Service is the most centralized among these industrialized nations. Operating since 1948, this universal system allows for the provision of a wide range of geographically accessible medical services. The National Health Service determines how much money to spend each year on health care by utilizing a capitation method for general physicians and a fee-for-service system for specialists. The general physician's role is that of 'gatekeeper', determining when and if a patient needs to see a specialist. This system has come under criticism because health care decisions are all too often based on the 'social utility' rather than the desire of the patient (i.e. older patients may be denied major surgery because they do not have many remaining productive years). However, these 'utilitarian attitudes' by physicians and policymakers, along with a fixed annual health care budget, enabled the U.K. to keep its percentage of GDP spent on health care to one of the lowest levels of all the industrialized nations (Graig, 1993).

Developed over 25 years ago, the Canadian health care system also offers universal coverage to all of its citizens along with portability of medical services from province to province. The federal government distributes funds to the ten provinces based on the size and wealth of their populations. Each province has a Ministry of Health that is the only payer of medical services. If a province spends more than what the federal government allocates to them, then the province must pay the difference on its own. Each provincial government and the medical care providers annually negotiate physician fees and hospital budgets. Most hospitals are not-for-profit organizations and patients can choose their own doctor in a fee-for-service arrangement.

Canadian health system

Canada's health care costs as a percentage of the GDP are kept at smaller levels than the United States by lower fees to physicians, hospitals and administrative personnel; and by uniformly distributing physicians in urban and rural areas so as to avoid geographic oversupply. Decreased use of capital intensive high technology items is another cost-saving device. High-technology equipment is usually only approved for use in specialized centers, and is closely controlled by the ministries of health in each province (Fulton, 1993).

Finally, developed in the 1920s, Japan's universal health care system receives financing from multiple sources: 60% from employed, 33% from self-employed and pensioners, and finally 7% from a special geriatric pool. The government strictly regulates reimbursement of medical services from prescription costs to physician fees, and thus allows Japan to spend a lower level of the GDP on health care. Japan's citizens have the highest life expectancy rate and the lowest infant mortality rate among the industrialized nations. Factors accounting for these exceptional rates vary. However, many experts attribute Japan's middle to upper socioeconomic status and diet as playing major roles. Also, Japan's prenatal care is deemed one of the

Japan's universal health care system

best, as Japan provides free and unlimited medical services to all pregnant women, infants and children. Pregnant women are educated in counseling classes and are visited by nurses and midwives in their homes. Japan's healthiness is remarkable, a sobering fact that the United States cannot ignore (Marmor, 1994).

Summary and Conclusions

Managed care came about from the pressure on employers to pay for the dramatic increases in health care insurance. Employers insisted that insurers and providers restrain health care inflation and at the same time provide comprehensive, continuing care to their employees.

The late 20th century also witnessed a greater percentage of Americans over age 65, and with that the accompanying problems of an aged population. While this over 65 age group comprises 15% of the current population, it is estimated by the year 2030 this group will account for 30%. Another factor affecting health care costs in the late 20th century are the changing disease patterns. Hypertension, hypertensive heart disease and various malignancies have continued to increase since 1970. The 1980s saw the development of HIV and AIDS that now claims victims in all strata of the population.

The increases in national health care expenditures, such as hospital services and long term care, as central to the expansion of managed care are presented. Hospital services represented the largest component of health care expenditures in 1994 – 36%, and the cost of long-term health care is sure to be a major hurdle given the aging U.S. population. In addition, this chapter presented the failed Clinton Health Security Act as well as innovative health care reforms proposed at the state level. Finally, an overview of the health financing structures of other industrialized nations was reviewed as a comparison to the United States.

3. Systems of Managed Care

Insurance, whether for health or home, is protection against an untoward event. By pooling small amounts of money from a larger population, risk is spread over many people. This concept of risk is essential in deciphering the maze of health care payment programs currently available. Presented in this chapter are various systems of managed health care that spread a shared financial risk between consumer and provider. Also, at the end of this chapter a fictional family will be introduced and followed through the decision-making process as they select a health plan to meet their needs. However, before discussing the various systems of managed care, it is important to review the traditional indemnity model.

For many years, the **indemnity health insurance** plan was the most common form of coverage in the United States and bore full risk for health care expenditures. This traditional model usually consists of an employer-paid premium to an insurance company, who then reimburses providers on a **fee-for-service** basis ('fee-for-service' also applies to services completely paid by the patient). **Providers** includes physicians and other individual health care providers, as well as hospitals, pharmacies or nursing homes. Sometimes, patients pay providers out-of-pocket and then receive reimbursement from the insurer (indemnity). An example of this type of plan is Blue Cross/Blue Shield. These indemnity plans usually reimburse the individual only a percentage of the incurred charge, typically 80%, and, in addition, most had annual deductibles that must be met before even the 80% of costs would be reimbursed.

Managed care elements were introduced in the 1970s into indemnity plans. Plans began to set fee schedules for provider reimbursements, so that the 80% reimbursement was no longer a percent-

indemnity health insurance

fee-for-service
Providers

age of the provider's charge, but of some predetermined **'usual, customary and reasonable' (UCR) fee** for a particular service. Today, few indemnity plans exist without some features of managed care, and such plans are only utilized by about 30% of the insured patient population (Field and Shapiro, 1995). Elements of managed care employed by indemnity plans include mental health benefits, precertification requirements for procedures or hospital admissions, and pharmaceutical benefits.

> **Managed health care** is a system of health care delivery that attempts to manage the cost and quality as well as the access to health care. Unique to this system is contracted providers who share in the financial risk of health care services, limitations to subscribers, and some type of authorization. Following are the spectrum of systems that comprise managed health care. These include: **Health Maintenance Organizations, Preferred Provider Organizations, Exclusive Provider Organizations, Point of Service Plans, Physician Hospital Organizations** and **Integrated Healthcare Systems.**

Health Maintenance Organizations (HMOs)

Health Maintenance Organizations (HMOs) are among the earliest of the managed care approaches to be introduced, as early as the 1930s. These health delivery systems provide comprehensive health care for a fixed, prepaid fee, and they represent a major effort to control supply and demand in the health care market. HMOs contract directly with health care service providers, including individual health practitioners and hospitals or other facilities. In some cases, HMOs directly employ providers, including physicians and other health care professionals, and may also own the facilities in which they operate. The HMO typically receives payment from employers for specific service provision to employees who have enrolled for this coverage.

members

primary care physician

gatekeeper model

HMOs then are responsible for delivery of health care to enrolled **members**. Patients who belong to the plan are typically required to enter the plan through a **primary care physician** and choose their providers from among those associated with the HMO. Frequently, this is referred to as the **'gatekeeper' model**. Thus, when an enrolled member becomes seriously ill, the HMO bears the cost. Providers who are paid a flat fee (e.g., monthly) may be at great fiscal risk under this system, which provides an incentive to control costs. Thus, the HMO approach demonstrates one of the key elements inherent in managed care: they control costs by putting providers in a position to lose money by extensive or inefficient treatment, or having an unusually sick population. It is interesting to note that by the end of 1995, an estimated 53 million Americans were enrolled in some type of HMO. fig. 3.1 illustrates that HMO enrollment has dramatically risen since 1976.

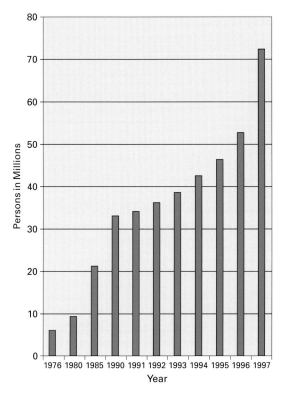

Fig. 3.1 HMO Enrollment

Source: Health, United States 1996–1997. National Center for Health Statistics.

Five basic models of HMOs are in operation: I the Independent Practice (Physician) Association (IPA); 2. the Group Model; 3. the Network Model; 4. the Staff Model; and 5. the Mixed Model. These models are now described in greater detail.

Independent Practice Association. The most common HMO arrangement, the Independent Practice (or Physician) Association (IPA*)* is an HMO that contracts with **licensed independent practitioners** in private practice or with independent associations of physicians or practices. In turn, the latter contract with their member practitioners. Examples of IPAs include HMO Blue in Massachusetts, Blue Choice in New York, and U.S. Healthcare, Inc., in New Jersey. Most IPA practitioners are also solo providers and thus they are likely to see a number of patients who are not members of the HMO as well. IPAs do not have medical facilities of their own (except their own offices), and provide care in the facilities of the independent provider, generally at a reduced (capitated or discounted) fee-for-service. All services are contracted, including hospitals and pharmaceuticals. A fund created from withheld providers' fees (typically about 20%) provides the HMO with a cushion against cost overruns, thereby managing cost containment. Such measures make practitioners aware of cost concerns. IPAs use typical managed care strategies, such as utilization review, management information systems, and centralized marketing and other administrative services.

Group Model. The Group Model HMO contracts with an independent practitioner group, usually with multiple specialties, to provide care to the HMO's members. Often the practitioner group provides care exclusively to the HMO membership; sometimes practitioners also see non-member patients. The HMO pays the group a member per month fee, (fixed or capitated), so the more a member uses services, the less the providers make. In some cases, group model HMOs pay direct costs to providers for services. Group Model HMOs frequently operate their own facilities, including hospitals, pharmacies, laboratories, and radiology services. The largest group model HMO, and one of the oldest, Kaiser Foundation Health Plan of Northern and Southern California regions, together served nearly five million members by the end of 1993.

Network Model. The Network Model HMO contracts with multiple practitioner groups, similar to the Group Model HMO, but without the exclusivity of a single provider group. By using more than one multi-specialty group, the HMO is able to offer a wider geographical coverage. Examples of Network Model HMOs are Blue Plus of Minnesota and TakeCare Health Plan of California. Unlike Group Model plans, the Network HMO does not usually own the facilities, but instead the practitioners or other contracted service providers supply the facilities, including pharmacies and hospitals. Sometimes, Network Model plans employ combinations of models; for example, staff models (see below) with some other form of delivery, such as a group or IPA model. The Network Model uses capitation with all providers. Members usually choose a primary care physician, however, providers are frequently able to see non-HMO patients in their practice.

Staff Model. Perhaps the easiest HMO arrangement to compre- hend is the Staff Model, a plan that employs providers on a salary and treats enrolled members in the HMO's own setting. Examples include Harvard Community Health Plan in Massachusetts and Humana Health Plan, Inc., in Florida. Like Group Model HMOs, these organizations often own and operate hospitals, laboratories, and other medical facilities, although this is not always the case. Some make contracts with community facilities and specialists outside the staff for services.

The high cost of building and maintaining facilities translates into a lack of growth for staff model HMO plans. Yet, in terms of cost-containment and efficient management, staff and group model plans tend to be the most effective.

Mixed Model. In the first decade after the HMO Act passed, when managed care began to explode, the various models were clearly defined. However, consolidation is occurring throughout the industry, so that several different models now merge under a larger umbrella organization. These arrangements, also termed 'networks', add to the confusion around definitions in this field. Mixed-Model HMOs are combinations of any of the first four models described above. As the field continues to expand, the hybrid models are becoming so common that the distinctions among the types of models described here are often difficult to identify. Nevertheless, fig. 3.2 shows the most recent breakdown of the various model types comprising HMO plans.

Because of the cost associated with staff and group models, the IPA model plans are the fastest-growing HMO plan, accounting for nearly 50% of all HMO membership, and more than half of all HMO plans. HMOs are most common in the West and Northeast. HMOs generally provide benefits which are comprehensive, including cradle-to-grave services such as prenatal, perinatal, and infant care, childhood immunizations, and annual physical examinations, as well as emergency care, hospitalization, physical therapy, mental health and

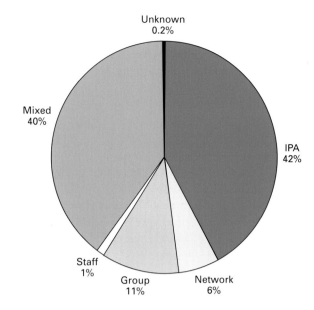

Fig. 3.2   Model Types as Percentage of HMO Plans

Source: Copyright © 1999 by American Association of Health Plans. Reproduced by permission from AAHP.

substance abuse services. Many HMOs cover organ transplants, depending on the specific organ involved and the condition for which it is required.

Preferred Provider Organization (PPO)

Preferred Provider Organizations (PPOs) represent a combination of the traditional indemnity, or fee-for-service plans and the HMO models. PPOs are partnerships among a panel of providers, such as health care professionals, hospitals, and other health services, who in turn contract with purchasers of health care; for example, employers or insurance companies. PPOs differ from HMOs in several ways: they are not prepaid plans; i, Subscribers are encouraged to use participating providers, but they are not required to use them; ii, Subscribers may see out-of-network providers, but usually will pay more to do so; iii, There is no primary physician who serves as a 'gatekeeper,' who must authorize **referrals** to other specialists or services; iv, There is no capitation and; v, PPOs do not assume any financial risk (risk is carried by the purchaser). Like HMOs, PPOs provide services at a lower cost to

referrals

Rickel and Wise

subscribers within a defined group. Providers see patients as needed, bill independently for services as they deliver, but follow a specified fee schedule established in the contract with the purchaser. They also agree to comply with utilization review guidelines in their provision of services in exchange for the preferred referral status with subscribers.

Reimbursement to providers varies in PPO arrangements. Some pay a percentage of 'usual, customary, and reasonable' (UCR) fees, judged to be the 'going rate' for a particular service in a specific geographical area. Sometimes, PPOs agree to a fee freeze for the first year, with annual increases tied to the consumer price index. Others establish a discount to be deducted from the provider's fee schedule. In some cases, a system called a 'resource-based relative value scale' (RBRVS) may be used to rank the value of the procedure to the patient and the purchaser, so that a more common, less complicated procedure (e.g., appendectomy) receives a lower rating, and a more complicated, less common service (e.g., heart bypass surgery) receives a higher ranking. These rankings are then multiplied by a monetary conversion factor to produce a schedule of fees (Kelch, Amos and Elden, 1992).

usual, customary, and reasonable fees

> PPOs are highly variable, but generally provide an intermediary delivery system capable of comprehensive coverage at a low cost to the patient. Employees generally will choose a PPO rather than an HMO, when a choice is allowed. Every state now offers PPO networks, and they are most prevalent in the Midwest and the Southeastern United States. In addition to employer and insurance company ownership, PPOs may also be under the ownership of physicians, hospital chains, and other large groups.

Exclusive Provider Organization (EPO)

Combining the features of HMOs and PPOs, **Exclusive Provider Organizations** (EPOs) limit services to network providers. An EPO does not cover out-of-network providers. In these systems, there is a great deal of quality and cost control, through the use of gatekeepers, a select group of providers, capitated fees, and utilization management.

Point-of-Service (POS)

A **Point-of-Service** (POS) plan, similar to a PPO, offers services to subscribers at a reduced cost through a network of participating healthcare providers. However, unlike PPOs, POS plans utilize a 'gatekeeper' primary care physician who must authorize the use of any other providers or services. Out-of-network benefits are usually even less than those allowed under a PPO. **Deductibles** and higher **co-payments** charged for out-of-network services provide incentives for patients to choose network providers. Also, it can be difficult to get reimbursement for out-of-network services in a timely manner.

deductibles
co-payments

Increasingly, HMOs offer hybrid plans that include Point-of-Service options to allow subscribers to seek services outside the HMO. The number of HMOs offering POS plans grew from 20% to 75% in the last four years. As in other POS arrangements, the higher costs associated with out-of-network providers discourage the use of outside services. These options are expensive for health care purchasers (e.g., employers) as well as for health plans. However, they are pleasing to consumers, who prefer the sense of having some choice in their health care services, whether or not they exercise it. Consumer advocates believe POS plans are worth the cost as they provide access to services that might not be routinely ordered (Adelson, 1997).

Physician–Hospital Organization (PHO)

In response to managed care pressures, physicians and hospitals in some cases are joining together to form **Physician–Hospital Organizations (PHOs)**. The PHO contracts with health care purchasers, such as insurance companies, employers, and even some HMOs, who in turn agree to use only PHO providers and facilities. Providers are often part of a PPO or an IPA, which then enters into an agreement with a local hospital, with each party to the agreement providing capital and sharing the financial risk. However, the healthcare payer also shares some of the risk. Comprehensive care is provided, and like an HMO, the PHO usually accepts a prepaid, capitated fee for patients.

Integrated Healthcare System (IHS)

An **Integrated Healthcare System** (IHS) is an organization that is integrated vertically so that it provides a variety of services on a continuum of care. Services may include prevention services, acute, chronic, and long-term care, behavioral medicine, annual examinations and diagnostic screening, laboratory, radiology and rehabilitation services. Total patient care is the goal of this type of system, which makes it more comprehensive than the PHO. Full integration of services lowers cost by increasing efficiency of health care delivery to larger numbers of patients. As yet, such fully integrated services are rare (e.g., Fallon Healthcare System in Massachusetts; Rush System for Health in Chicago), but viewed by many as a goal for future service delivery.

Specialty HMOs and PPOs

Specialty managed care systems provide one or more limited health care benefits, such as pharmacy, vision, mental health, dental, oncology, chiropractic or Workers' Compensation. Specialty HMOs may be based on any of the five models described above. Specialty PPOs are similar to the PPOs described above for general health care.

Specialty Example: Mental Health. Based on the idea that mental health care is different from medical care and, thus, needs to be managed differently, health care payers (e.g., employers or insurance companies) increasingly turn to 'carving out' mental health benefits through **managed behavioral health care organizations**. Used with many specialty plans, **'Carve-outs'**, such as dental benefits (see also the pharmacy example below), indicate the separation of a specialty benefit from the broader medical plan. A carve-out may separate funding, design, delivery, certification procedures, utilization review, case management, claims reimbursement, and administrative functions from the broader medical coverage. Provider networks are separate as well, with utilization review personnel who have expertise in the carved-out specialty, and a unique set of co-payments, deductibles and limitations (Rubin, 1992).

managed behavioral health care organizations

Carve-outs

Some believe carve-outs are particularly well suited to mental health benefits, because of the distinctive nature of behavioral problems, the unique treatment plans required for individual patients and the need for reviewers to understand the particulars of mental health treatment. Cost containment is a major factor in a carve-out approach, allowing payers to offer more benefits and treatment options while controlling the provider source to keep costs under control. Although there are a number of advantages to carve-out arrangements, particularly for payers concerned with controlling cost, there are disadvantages as well. The latter include concerns that separating mental from medical care decreases co-ordination and integration of services, at a time when Americans are beginning to fully appreciate the interaction between mental and physical disorders, and when integrated services are considered the better approach to treating the whole patient in his/her community (Goodman, Brown and Dietz, 1992). One such example is the **day treatment center**. Among other advantages cited by supporters of the carve-out approach include the emphasis on family systems treatment, oversight of psychotropic medication use and co-ordination with Employee Assistance Programs (EAPs).

day treatment center

Specialty Example: Pharmacy. Under the traditional indemnity system, insurance companies used the prescription card for pharmacy benefits for some time. Although considered an unmanaged benefit (i.e., one without a cost-containment strategy and lacking systematic processing), these prescription card systems involve a co-payment, which is a low-fixed, pre-arranged, fee (usually less than ten dollars) paid by the consumer at the point of sale. The insurer reimburses the pharmacy for the actual cost of the substance, plus a dispensing fee to cover administrative costs of filling in the prescription and submitting a claim. Co-payments are not generally subject to a deductible. The availability of these cards led to greater use of prescription services, thus leading to the problem of cost control.

pharmacy benefits

To provide better cost containment, health care payers (e.g., employers or insurance companies) are carving out pharmacy benefits, similar to the carve-outs described for mental health. To control the costs of prescription benefits, managed care introduced a number of strategies. Among the most commonly used approaches are the development of formularies, substitution of generic compounds and prior authorization.

formularies

Formularies are a major component of managed care pharmacy services. While open formularies allow reimbursement for all prescriptions, with virtually no control or limits placed on prescribers, closed formularies save at least 10% on medications and are thus favored by managed care. A closed formulary lists specific drugs reimbursed under a health plan and organizes the drugs by their therapeutic class. In addition to cost alone, the efficacy and safety of drugs are important in a plan's decision to list them in a formulary.

Generic substitutions evolved from the managed care trend of see- generic substitutions
king lower cost services, use of electronic processing, and contracted
services with pharmacies, either retail chains or those operated by
plans. Generic medications are often cheaper, 40 to 70%, than brand-
name drugs. In HMOs, about 40% of prescriptions are filled with gene-
rics, and about two-thirds of HMOs require generic substitution whenever possible. The largest HMOs, as well as those with the staff
model, are the most likely to utilize these policies and to practice them.

Yet another strategy affecting prescribers is the use of **prior au-** prior authorization
thorization requirements for specific drugs. This approach allows
managed care organizations to control the use of certain medications,
but it places the decision for their need or appropriateness in the
hands of managed care case managers, taking it out of the hands of
the provider. This changes the dynamics of patient care, forcing the
health care professional that examined the patient face-to-face to
relinquish authority over some aspects of his/her treatment. Authorization numbers must be obtained from the case manager to be entered onto the prescription form before the prescription may be filled,
if it is to be covered by the payer. Given the increasingly high costs
of medication, compared to patient co-payments, this is a strong
incentive for the patient to adhere to the insurer's regulations.

Employee Assistance Programs (EAPs)

Several decades ago, **Employee Assistance Programs** (EAPs)
developed as in-house divisions where employees could talk about
work problems. Many of these evolved into centers for substance
abuse counseling, but in recent years, EAPs developed into programs
for screening and referral, and some time-limited counseling, for a
range of mental health problems (Masi and Caplan, 1992). EAPs are
growing in popularity, as they save money for companies. They also
became increasingly attractive to independent practitioners attemp-
ting to adapt to the changing marketplace.

The major goal of EAPs is to enhance productivity by decreasing the need for workers to take leave from work because of mental health stresses. A number of studies demonstrated the cost-effectiveness of the EAP approach. The typical cost to employers is about
$20 to $30 per employee, but potential savings for the large employer can be in the millions in terms of the reduction in insurance claims
and in time lost from work. Recent surveys of EAPs indicate about
80% of the companies with more than 1,000 workers offer EAPs. For

smaller companies (larger than 50 employees), about a third offer EAPs to workers.

Integrated Services: 'Seamless Garments' of Care

As described in this chapter, managed care is a collection of components, managed by several different individuals, such as benefits managers, utilization reviewers and providers. Key to the successful operation of this system is skillful communication among the various elements, so that co-ordinated efforts allow patients to experience prompt and effective treatment, which is optimally economical yet, high in quality. Some compare this goal to the image of the 'seamless garment', where integrated service delivery provides comprehensive, cradle-to-grave coverage to recipients, who are unaware of the complexity of the interactions required for all components to work together smoothly in the delivery of these services.

For some time, managed care organizations and academic medical centers (AMCs) appeared to be hopelessly at odds, with managed care's emphasis on primary care gatekeepers, cost-cutting, and decreased use of specialists, against AMCs training and promotion of medical specialties, and trial-and-error experimentation with new methods and techniques for treatment.

Nevertheless, this vision of a future with managed care as a permanent part of the landscape is reflected in a number of attempts to begin integration of medical training and managed care systems. So far, these arrangements primarily involve HMOs joining forces with AMCs, with both groups recognizing the need to better prepare health care professionals to operate in the managed care environment (Institute of Medicine, 1996).

Yet, public policy decisions, such as cuts to Medicare funding which formerly helped subsidize medical education, and the relentless growth of managed care, despite providers' trepidation, acted as a catalyst to AMCs' willingness to work with managed care to better prepare their graduates to function in the changing health care environment. At the same time, HMOs became more interested in training medical professionals, encouraging rotations in their facilities. Not only do new practitioners enter the marketplace better informed about the realities of managed care, but they also provide HMOs with a source of potential new hires.

In fact, such partnerships are not new, although they only recently began to multiply. For two decades, the Kaiser Foundation Health Plan of Northern and Southern California, with about five million members, trains its health care professionals. Medical students from Stanford University and two University of California medical schools rotate through Kaiser facilities. Below we describe some of the other partnerships that formed in recent years.

Harvard Medical School and Harvard Pilgrim Health Care. In 1992, Harvard Medical School (HMS) and the Boston-based HMO Harvard Pilgrim Health Care (HPHC) created a unique arrangement, they established the first medical school department located in an HMO facility (Moore, Inui, Ludden and Schoenbaum, 1994). The Department of Ambulatory Care and Prevention, established at HPHC yet part of HMS, created a 'teaching HMO', similar to a teaching hospital. Moore et al., cite six characteristics that describe the potential advantages of such a collaboration: 1. a new, academically affiliated department created a high-status entity with a new mission; 2. enhancement of the attractiveness of the HMO to potential new hires, as well as the possibility of career development for existing staff; 3. intensified interactions between faculty and trainees in real world settings where preventive medicine and health promotion approaches can be learned first-hand; 4. enhanced research opportunities by the presence of academic investigators and the access to clinical populations; 5. the HMO as a stable funding source provides needed security for medical school training; and 6. administrative efficiency established in the HMO is seen as a benefit to the encouragement of research efforts, as well as to a favorable teaching atmosphere.

Case Western Research University and Henry Ford Health System. In a somewhat unique arrangement, the School of Medicine at Case Western Reserve University (CWRU), located in Cleveland, joined in an alliance with the Henry Ford Health System (HFHS), located in Detroit, nearly 200 miles away (Stevens, Leach, Warden and Cherniack, 1996). HFHS, an integrated health care system serving more than three-quarters of a million patients, more than half of them part of a managed care plan (Health Alliance Plan), has a tradition of medical school training. For two decades, HFHS provided rotations for medical students from the University of Michigan, as well as a large number of house staff residents and fellows. HFHS wanted to affiliate with CWRU in order to establish a firmer collaboration with a medical school, and CWRU sought to enhance their students training in the managed care environment while expanding their opportunities for exposure to **ambulatory care** settings. Despite difficulties with different institutional cultures, territorial issues, and competitive concerns, the affiliation gained from shared commitments to education, research, training of students in managed care issues, and the value of a student presence in a medical setting. Stevens et al., conclude that the return has been worth the investment, from the perspective of both sides of the affiliation.

TennCare: University of Tennessee, and Meharry Medical College. Unlike the collaborative efforts described above, Tennessee's AMCs faced a rather sudden penetration of managed care into the health care system when the state turned its Medicaid recipients and other uninsured residents over to managed care organizations.

In 1993, the federal government took back $120 million in Medicaid funds from Tennessee, charging the state improperly administered federal matching requirements (Meyer and Blumenthal, 1996). In response to this fiscal crisis, Tennessee's governor, who was about to leave office, instituted TennCare, which put all the state's former Medicaid recipients under managed care, as well as all other state residents whose incomes were at or below the poverty line. The state also offered the option of purchasing this coverage, at a sliding-scale rate, to residents who were above the poverty line by up to 400%.

Meyer and Blumenthal (1996) studied the effects of this rapid implementation of a managed care system with nearly 25% of the state's population on two AMCs, the University of Tennessee Medical School (UT) and Meharry Medical College (MMC). The authors reviewed documents, conducted site visits, and interviewed AMC staff and management, state officials, and managed care representatives.

Both medical settings experienced large losses of revenue, closed some specialty services, reduced training positions (because of declining funds for medical education), lost patient populations needed for clinical research, and witnessed a shift in patient population mix towards a sicker population needing more expensive care (which now was reimbursed at a significantly lower rate). Meyer and Blumenthal (1996) concluded the consequences of such public-sector driven changes are similar to those experienced in the private sector.

On the other hand, Meyer and Blumenthal (1996) suggested there may be a potential for more positive outcomes, similar to the experiences of the voluntary collaborations described above. These include integration of community-based service with the AMC mission, increasingly diversified clinical services, and the opportunity to train students and residents in the realities of the managed care environment.

Kaiser Permanente and Georgetown University. The latest innovative collaboration between managed care and an AMC is the newly created program of Kaiser Permanente and Georgetown University Medical Center. Kaiser Permanente, the largest managed care organization in the country, has seven million enrolled members and employs 9,000 physicians nationwide. Since 1980, Kaiser Permanente controlled the Georgetown University Health Plan. Georgetown University, a leader in medical training, has in recent years increased collaborative efforts with Kaiser.

Recent joint ventures included monthly block electives in primary care at Kaiser, 'mini-sabbaticals' by Kaiser physicians to update their knowledge and skills at Georgetown, the use of Kaiser sites for off-campus practice opportunities for residents, and the institution of a primary care-internal medicine fellowship for post-residency training of internal medicine physicians in the managed, primary care environment of an HMO.

Discussions between Kaiser and Georgetown originally encompassed the integration of training in internal medicine. This led to the identification of a need for a training program that would integrate training in pediatrics and internal medicine. This merger of pediatrics and medicine training was the ideal training for providing the primary care skills necessary for physicians operating in a family and community-oriented HMO environment.

The two organizations set about designing a four-year medicine-pediatrics residency program with a dedicated site in the Kaiser Permanente system. The initial plan calls for 16 residents. However, once the training module develops, the expectation is that the program may become more widely used within the Kaiser system. Key elements of the curriculum and training experiences expect to become part of residency training in both traditional pediatrics and traditional medicine programs.

Finally, the Kaiser and Georgetown medicine-pediatrics residency generated a model curriculum and model training experiences that could be used nationally in generalist training programs. Training modules include instruction in family-centered primary care, managed care practice, ethical issues, and **quality assessment** and **quality improvement**.

quality assessment, quality improvement

Summary and Conclusions

This chapter traced the development of health care coverage in the United States from its beginnings as the traditional indemnity health insurance plan to today's emphasis on managed care systems. The five primary models of Health Maintenance Organizations (HMOs) were reviewed: 1. the Independent Practice Association (IPA); 2. the Group Model; 3. the Network Model; 4. the Staff Model; and 5. the Mixed Model. The latter model grew in recent years, as hybrid models combining the various types of provider networks are increasingly popular in response to market demands.

Another combination, the Preferred Provider Organization (PPO), blends elements of the traditional indemnity model with HMO characteristics, and the Exclusive Provider Organization (EPO) in turn brings together elements of PPOs with HMO features. Point-of-Service (POS) plans offer yet another approach to managed care, employing a 'gatekeeper' primary care physician that authorizes the use of any other providers or services.

Also, this chapter discussed organizational structures, such as the Physician-Hospital Organizations (PHOs) and the Integrated Healthcare Systems (IHSs), as well as introducing the concept of Specialty HMOs and PPOs. This chapter described specialty examples of 'carved-out' services for mental health and pharmacy benefits, as well as the increasing use of Employee Assistance Programs (EAPs). Also included in this chapter was the goal of a 'seamless' delivery system, followed by several examples of collaborative efforts at integrating academic medical centers with managed care organizations, and the mutual benefits envisioned or realized from such integrative endeavors. Finally, the last part of the chapter outlined a newly formed collaboration that creates a new residency program and has the potential to influence medical training nationwide. As managed care appears to be a permanent part of the health care landscape, the elements described in this chapter will continue to be dynamic models that shift and change with the marketplace. Traditional divisions among practitioners, hospitals, and payers will become increasingly blurred. Limited resources and public policy decisions will continue to influence health care management, delivery and integration for years to come.

Now, to the case study of the Symington family. This fictional family will be followed as it moves to a new community and is offered various health plan options. By incorporating information learned in this chapter, the reader needs to problem-solve the most beneficial health plan for this family. The authors propose a choice and provide the rational for this decision.

Case Study of the Symington Family

This fictional family consists of:

Michael Symington
age 43
manager of supermarket
suffers from lower back pain

Kathy Symington
age 40
employed part-time as a librarian
pre-cancerous breast disease

Ricky Symington
age 13
student in 8th grade
bronchial asthma since age 3

Renee Symington
age 10
student in 5th grade
excellent health

Background Information

The Symingtons recently moved to the East Coast where Michael accepted a position as a store manager for a large supermarket chain. Michael's previous position was as a store manager with a small independent market, and he lost his health insurance benefits when he left that position. Michael's health insurance coverage at his new company is not in effect yet. Thus, Michael pays out-of-pocket for his family's medical care and therefore the family does not receive the attention they require. For example, Ricky Symington is not taking all of his prescribed asthma medication because they cannot afford it, Kathy Symington is unable to see the specialist that she was referred to by her Doctor in the Midwest who had identified her precancerous breast condition, and Michael did not seek treatment for his lower back problems. Michael chose to work for a large food chain since he knew he would be offered several health plan options. Michael is anxious to meet with the insurance benefits representative to review his benefits options based on his family's health care coverage needs.

When Michael meets with the employee health benefits representative, he learns that his legal spouse and dependent children under age 19 are eligible for health care coverage. According to IRS rules, Michael can only change his coverage for health care when a change in his family's status occurs. These changes in status can include the following: divorce or legal separation of a spouse; birth or adoption of a child; addition of a dependent; death of a spouse or dependent; or an employment status change for Michael or his wife Kathy.

The company offers Michael the following options of health insurance plans:

1. A Traditional Indemnity Model

- free choice of providers
- $175 monthly premium for a family
- $600 annual deductible per family
- 20% co-pay per office visit/hospitalization
- No prescription drug coverage

2. A Preferred Provider Organization

Within the Provider Network
- No deductibles
- $15 co-pay per office visit
- $45 co-pay per ER visit
- $10 co-pay per prescriptions

Outside the Provider Network
- $350 annual deductible
- $25 co-pay per office visit
- $85 co-pay per ER visit
- $10 co-pay per prescriptions
- $120 monthly premium for a family

3. An HMO Health Plan

Mixed Model Network

- Choice limited to approved network providers – can switch freely within plan
- No deductibles or co-pays
- $85 monthly premium for a family
- $5 co-pay per prescription

Which plan should Michael choose for his family?

Michael needs to weigh the various health plan options based on his financial capabilities as well as his family's medical coverage needs.

In the Traditional Plan, the Symingtons can select any health care provider, including a specialist, but there would be high out-of-pocket expenses along with high premiums, deductibles and co-pays. There would be no coverage for prescription drugs such as asthma medication, which it appears Ricky Symington needs on a continuing basis.

In the Preferred Provider Organization Plan the Symingtons have some flexibility in choosing health care services. There are no deductibles if the Symingtons stay within the provider network, however, they are responsible for any amounts in excess of the covered charges charged by an out-of-network provider. There are co-pays required for outpatient treatments and prescription drugs but monthly premiums are less expensive than the Traditional Plan. Each member of the family must select a primary care physician from the provider directory, and numerous hospitals in the area are part of the network.

The Health Maintenance Organization plan limits freedom to choose health care providers, however there are no deductibles or co-pays and a lower monthly premium. There is only a $5 co-pay for prescription drugs purchased from a participating pharmacy. The Symingtons can only receive care through a network provider, with the exception of life threatening emergency treatment. This plan covers hospitalization services only with area hospitals affiliated with the HMO plan and the plan also covers preventive care.

Given the health history of the Symingtons, their use of medical as well as surgical services could be significant. Therefore, Michael decides to join the HMO plan because it has a full range of primary care, specialty and preventive care services at a manageable financial cost to him.

4. Components of a Managed Care System

Within the growing revolution that currently defines health care in the United States, managed care partially developed in response to the demands for both organization and delivery of medical services. The overall aims of managed care systems, regardless of structure, are to reduce or eliminate unnecessary services and reduce the cost of health care. While pursuing these objectives, the quality of treatment is presumably not reduced. Because these organizations are able to achieve large cost savings, they have become attractive to both employers and patients, and thus, increased in size. Managed care is so prevalent that 85% of the U.S. working population is in some form of network as reported by the William M. Mercer benefits consulting firm (Freudenheim, 1998).

Managed care has certain common elements, although plans may take a variety of forms. Managed care plans establish networks of service providers who agree to the conditions of a contract and choose providers based on the cost, quality and range of services they provide. Access to a plan is often through a 'gate-keeper' or single point of entry, a primary care provider. The primary care provider usually manages patient access to specialists and other plan service providers. In addition, the managed care plans shift financial risk to service providers by a variety of reimbursement systems. One payment method is a capitation contract that prepays the provider a set monthly amount for each enrollee. In return, the provider agrees to provide services for that set amount. Discounted rates and fee schedules are other payment methods that are sometimes used

(Kongstvedt, 1997). The following chapter gives an overview of the essential components of a managed care system. Also, at the end of the chapter, the case study of the Symington family continues as they confront various health problems which require medical attention.

Contracted Provider Network

multidisciplinary credentialing

A managed care organization contracts with both primary care and specialty providers, often solo practitioners, to develop a network of **multidisciplinary** credentialed clinicians. The **credentialing** of the providers involves a review process to determine if the individual possesses an unrestricted state license, is board certified if appropriate, and holds current malpractice insurance. The multidisciplinary nature of a behavioral health care provider network might involve for example: adult and child psychiatrists and psychologists, addictionologists, psychiatric nurse specialists, and social workers. The network diversifies the providers by rationing for each discipline.

partial hospitalization

Also included in the network of services are the various facilities that aim to provide an 'integrated health care system' or 'seamless' care under one organizational umbrella. An integrated health care system includes: inpatient facilities which provide acute and long-term care in general and psychiatric hospitals, as well as residential treatment centers; **partial hospitalization** and day treatment services which provide clinical services as an alternative or follow-up to inpatient hospital care; outpatient programs which range from ambulatory care centers that provide outpatient surgery to routine office based care, and home based care, the newest area of service, which involves the provision of health care within a patient's home by medically supervised professionals. Patients at home can receive numerous treatments for acute or long-term illnesses such as cancer, and at a much lower cost.

These integrated health care networks through the process of buyouts and mergers will dominate health care in the 21st Century. Fears that they will have no enrollees or patients are making physicians, hospitals, and insurance companies consolidate their operations. In fact, many states are passing legislation to form these networks. Eight hospitals in St. Louis, Missouri formed an integrated delivery network in 1993, and in Kansas City, Missouri a for-profit network formed merging the hospital system of Health Midwest, Providence Medical Center, two other hospitals and Blue Cross/Blue

Shield (Bodenheimer and Grumbach, 1995). While merging these systems may not initially result in 'seamless' continuity, it is sometimes necessary if these various entities are to survive.

Patient Access Systems

Ideally, patients should have immediate access to clinicians by phone or in person on a 24-hour basis. However, frequently a primary care physician or family practitioner co-ordinates patient care, usually through a single 'gatekeeper' physician. Sometimes the 'gatekeeper' can be an internist, a pediatrician, an osteopathic physician, or a nurse practitioner. These 'gatekeepers' initially treat the patient and make decisions about their risk level, problem type and subsequent referrals (Cassell, 1997). Each patient is **triaged**, a term that refers to a military procedure that determines who is at highest risk and is most in need of services. For example, if it were an emergency situation, the doctor would recommend treatment in an inpatient facility, while for more routine situations the doctor would recommend treatment on an outpatient basis.

triaged

The risk level and problem type of the patient determines the discipline of the treating clinician. For example, in the case of a suicidal patient on anti-depressant medication, the clinician recommended would be a physician.

Geographic and demographic patient requests are honored if feasible. When a patient speaks only Spanish and requests a clinician who understands that language, such a request is given a high priority.

Utilization Management/Case Management

This process attempts to co-operatively integrate the review and management of health care services with all parties involved (e.g., providers, patients, employers and payers) (Boland, 1992). Most insurance plans today use **utilization management** techniques or **treatment planning** procedures. Utilization management refers to the evaluation and determination of the **appropriateness** of patient use of medical resources, and provision of any needed assistance to clinician and/or member, to ensure appropriate use of resources. These include **prior authorization** for hospital admission or the intended procedures as well as pre-admission certification for inpatient treatment based on anticipated length of stay and established

utilization management
treatment planning
appropriateness

prior authorization

medical criteria. In addition, a patient's care is monitored concurrently during an emergency or while undergoing treatment. Managed care plans conduct **retrospective reviews** after treatment to audit the quality of the procedures and to check for indications of unnecessary use of services (Corcoran and Vandiver, 1996).

Managed care organizations also use **practice guidelines** to determine the appropriateness and the medical necessity of care. These guidelines are systematically developed outcome-based statements on the proper procedures for specific medical conditions. The main objectives of these guidelines are to improve patient care, limit inappropriate procedures, reduce unwanted variation, and maintain cost efficiency. Several entities developed guidelines, including the **Agency for Health Care Policy and Research (AHCPR)** of the U.S. Department of Health and Human Services, medical societies, and pharmaceutical manufacturers.

AHCPR was instrumental in determining guidelines for treating acute pain which hospitals widely accepted and led them to adopt aggressive postoperative pain management programs. However, at this time there are approximately 1,500 practice guidelines developed and distributed by over 45 agencies and organizations. Thus, before a managed care organization makes a decision regarding which practice guidelines to use, they may need to convene their medical leadership with experts in the field. Nevertheless, providers associated with multiple managed care plans may be confronted with different guidelines for treating the same disease. In this case the health care professional may use these guidelines as a set of practice options and not as a standard of treatment.

Case management, another utilization management program, involves using health care resources in an efficient and cost effective manner. Case management is the process of identifying patients at risk for high cost care and for facilitating the development and implementation of appropriate care. For example, with regard to discharge planning, questions a case manager addressed include: What is the appropriate time that a patient is ready to be discharged from the hospital? What needs to be in place for the patient as they move to the next level of care in order to eliminate or reduce the need for unnecessary treatment? If a patient has a chronic condition, has payment for this care been authorized? The case manager constructs linkages between elements of a treatment plan and community services to provide a 'continuum of care' while serving as patient advocate and provider advisor.

Group practices with delegated or internal review are a new direction that managed care companies are pursuing. This involves the formation of multidisciplinary group practices that take back the utilization management/case management responsibilities from the managed care organization after having proven their efficiency and effectiveness.

Claims Payment/Fiscal Controls

This procedure is increasingly becoming an electronic process and eventually everything will be paperless. It is important that providers and managed care organizations have sophisticated information systems in place in order that authorizations for treatment and **claims** processing are handled efficiently. Currently, some settings already institute Electronic Data Interchange (EDI), a standard methodology of exchanging information across organizations. While not fully developed by health care industry, future applications for EDI propose such advances as an ATM Swipe Card, which would include patient medical records and payment records (Traska, 1992).

One of the purposes of paying claims is to enable the managed care organization to have fiscal control over patients and providers. The managed care organization encourages cost-consciousness through channeling patients to the most cost-efficient providers and to the suitable level of care. Managed care organizations use incentives to keep costs down (i.e., in some plans smaller co-payments are required if generic drugs are selected over brand-names).

In the case of providers, claims data enables the managed care organization to identify and deal with high spending providers as well as quality and cost-efficient providers (Pauly, Eisenberg and Radany, 1992). Referred to as profiling, this process focuses on the patterns of an individual provider's care. A provider's profile is compared to a peer group or a **standard** and is used to measure performance and to guide quality improvements. For instance, high spending providers might be dealt with in several ways. **Capitation** of the provider is one method used by the managed care organization. That is, a per capita rate is usually paid monthly to the provider who is then responsible for delivering all health services required by the patients in a managed care plan. An example would be a family practitioner that would receive $20,000 per month to cover all health care costs for his 1,000 patients. Suspending referrals without necessarily informing the provider is another method for dealing with high-cost providers, also increasing the intensity of their review is yet another way of dealing with them.

claims

standard

Capitation

Also, some managed care plans send clinicians **'report cards'** altering them to areas where they did not follow plan policy or where their practices deviated from those of their peers.

Customer Service

Managed care companies approach **customer service** in two ways, one is oriented toward the consumer, and the other is toward the provider. A member or purchaser of a managed care plan often has numerous questions concerning the rules and procedures of the plan despite written material provided. Therefore, a member can telephone the managed care organization directly concerning such issues as eligibility and available benefits. These questions might involve 'How does one get certified for treatment?' or 'How many outpatient visits are available for mental health treatment?' Sometimes inquiries may involve determining information concerning what doctors are in the network or are **grievances** about not wanting to be treated by the referred provider.

Claims and appeals make up a final category of member questions. The **appeals mechanism** is a formal process that the provider of service and/or a member can use to request review of a plan decision. Often, members ask why a claim hasn't been paid, or appeal a claim which was paid at a lesser amount than submitted.

Clinicians also approach managed care organizations with a myriad of questions. Sometimes a doctor may have 50 patients, each with a different benefit plan. Therefore, it is imperative that the managed care organization provides program information to the doctor regarding a specific patient's benefits.

Payment issues such as late payment or non-payment are also frequent reasons that clinicians contact a managed care organization. Lastly, a clinician often questions their network status. They may have recently applied to a managed care panel and haven't heard regarding acceptance or have recently received a probation/termination letter. These situations all require contact with the managed care organization to determine ones' status.

With regard to paying the provider, many managed care companies pay their bills relatively promptly, with the average payment being 54 days. However, some of the slowest payers include some of the biggest HMOs, as can be seen in fig. 4.1. What are the reasons for these delays? Executives from some of the biggest HMOs state that the numbers are misleading. They insist that time-consuming

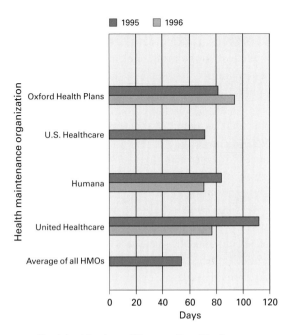

Fig. 4.1   Number of Days to Pay Vendor
Source: New York Times, April 17, 1997. From Company Reports; Interstudy.

paperwork and upgrading their computer systems lead to payment delays in the past, as these companies struggled to keep up with the ever-increasing caseload as a result of mergers and burgeoning contracts. However, they now state that the 'kinks' are gone so that late payments are no longer an issue (Freudenheim, 1997).

Quality Management

Quality of care is the issue of the moment and involves the activities and programs in a managed care organization that provide confidence that patient care will satisfy stated requirements. To ensure quality and **accountability**, critical stakeholders in the health care market are demanding that managed care plans provide credible evidence of high levels of patient satisfaction and perceptible improvements in health status. A recent study published in the Journal of the American Medical Association by the New England Medical Center raised controversy and concern among the public regarding the quality of care they receive under managed care. The study followed 2,235 chronically ill patients from age 18 to 97 for four years, and

Quality of care

accountability

concluded that managed care is inferior care for the poor and elderly. In addition, the study found managed care best served a young, healthy, and financially well off population (Zelman, 1996).

performance
measurement

Performance measurement is one area of quality management and provides information on fundamental domains, (e.g., in the administrative area, how quickly are claims paid and customer problems resolved; in the financial area, is medical spending in line with the health care plans' income?).

clinical outcomes

A second area in quality management involves **clinical outcomes**. Measures selected determine the significance of disorders in terms of prevalence, morbidity and mortality and provide outcome data on services and procedures. Measures with reliability and validity ideally would be employed that do not place a burden on data providers. Further, empirical evidence should link the measures to health outcome and conform to U.S. public health objectives. For example, treatment processes need to be determined. What is the setting, frequency and type of treatment utilized as well as treatment results (how well are patients doing at the conclusion of treatment and at follow-up)?

Network outcomes are a third area of consideration in the quality management area. A managed care organization should annually review providers' credentials for recredentialling and should routinely conduct site reviews. Managed care organization's perceived practice by some consumer groups of paying incentives to physicians to restrict necessary care is coming under intense scrutiny. President Clinton's 20-person Healthcare Commission comprised of representatives from labor, state governments, consumers, providers and insurers is focusing on 'consumer protection' and 'quality' in managed care. Unacceptable plan practices, such as 'drive-through deliveries', and 'drive-through mastectomies', where patients' hospital stays are limited to 24 hours, have led to this **oversight**.

In the State of the Union Address delivered by President Clinton on January 27, 1998, he reiterated the urgency for Congress to pass the Health Consumer Bill of Rights. With a staggering 160 million citizens enrolled in managed care plans, he believes it is vital that they understand all their medical options, not just the least expensive. Furthermore, President Clinton stated that people should have the right to choose the doctor they want for the care they need; they should have the right to emergency room care whenever they need it; and they should have the right to keep their medical records confidential (Clinton, 1998).

consumer rights bills

There are also various models of comprehensive consumer rights bills being proposed in state legislatures. For instance, lawmakers in Florida stepped in to readjust the balance of power between patients and managed care plans. State law now makes it easier for patients to go to emergency rooms without worrying about whether their HMO will pay the bill. Also, patients have the right to be informed about expensive treatments and be heard by an outside board if their health plan refuses to pay for their care (Goldstein, 1998).

In addition, the American Medical Association developed the Patient Protection Act that establishes standards for managed care organizations. These standards address consumer benefits, access, and appeal's processes. The Managed Care Consumer Bill of Rights is another consumer-based approach promoted by the Citizens Fund that addresses such areas as geographic access to providers, choice of providers and patient protection clauses.

Women in Government developed a unique Managed Care Consumer Protection Act. Most noteworthy in this Act are provisions requiring managed care plans to use a 'prudent lay person' definition of emergency care and cover that care without prior authorization; to include performance measures and clinical outcomes data, and require managed care plans to develop a grievance and appeals process (American Nurses Association, 1997). Finally, more than 600,000 mental health professionals developed the Principals for the Provision of Mental Health and Substance Abuse Treatment Service which most importantly guarantees the protection of confidentiality in the therapist-client relationship except when law or ethics dictates otherwise.

A fourth, and final, area of quality management involves internal or external audits. A managed care organization sometimes conducts an internal audit itself or hires external auditors to assess performance.

> audits

Managed care organizations should understand their requirements and therefore should develop measurements toward fully meeting or exceeding those requirements. In this increasingly competitive health care environment with tighter and tighter profit margins, such measures provide the basis for comparing the value of competing health plans.

Future Directions

Managed care organizations will control the health care delivery system for the foreseeable future. However, the issue of 'quality' will most likely become the playing field in which significant changes will be disputed. These changes will be driven by consumer health concerns and satisfaction, as well as technical and professional outcomes of care.

Another area that will also receive significant attention in the near future will be capitation. It is estimated that by the year 2005, about 50% of the United States population will be covered by a capitated plan (Ruskin, 1997). Capitation allows both providers as well as managed care organizations to share in the financial risk, thus giving providers more reason to make more cost conscious decisions when treating their patients. The ethics of quality care become heatedly debated as financial incentives may lead the physician to provide insufficient, substandard treatment in order to meet their capitation requirements. However, it is equally important to question whether managed care organizations will interfere with physician decision making as a result of capitation.

Does the managed care organization influence the provider in such a way to help him adjust to his reduced income? Will future trends mean that managed care organizations train providers to practice in a capitated environment? Will the managed care organization provide practice guidelines to assist providers in helping them to stay within their budgets? These are all important questions to consider as capitation becomes a solution to the significant problems facing today's managed care industry.

per patient vs. global capitation

Currently, there are two types of capitation: one pays a capitiated sum per patient to individual providers, while the other capitation is considered 'global', where payers (such as corporate employers) pay a flat fee per enrollee annually and thus the health plan assumes the financial risk for the enrollee's care (Morreim, 1997). Future trends indicate that global capitation is a concept that multispecialty groups can embrace with encouraging outcomes. Global capitation means that providers alone do not assume all the financial risk of patient care and instead will be part of a larger health plan that allots a specified sum for their services. So, the health plan can use this large pot of money in whatever ways work best to provide inpatient and outpatient care to its patients with greater flexibility and freedom (Morreim, 1997).

disease-state management

An approach to health care that continues to undergo change is **disease-state management** (Todd and Nash, 1997). It begins with preventive health care and aggressive screening programs to detect diseases as early as possible. Disease specific practice guidelines are built into computer models that practitioners can use to assist them in patient treatment planning. Ideally, the managed care plan tracks a patient with a chronic disorder from an outpatient setting through

continuity of care

the health care system so as to achieve **continuity of care** and secure suitable treatment at each stage of the disease. There is an instructional component of the package, as well as providing educational materials to patients and families regarding the disease and strategies to enhance patient compliance.

Steps to optimize patient compliance enhance treatment outcomes because costly complications of some diseases can be prevented. For example, making sure that patients comply with therapeutic regimens can prevent the macrovascular and microvascular complications of poorly controlled diabetes. Other diseases in which early detection and appropriate treatment can avoid costly interventions later on include: ulcers, asthma, depression, hypertension and cardiovascular disease.

An additional technique of medical decision-making is **evidence-based medicine**. A leader in this movement is the Center for Evidence-Based Medicine in Oxford, England. Physicians search databases for sound medical research to determine tests and treatments evaluated with randomized controlled trials. Instead of a physician treating a patient based on what they have always done, evidence-based medicine recommends treatment for a patient based on large research trials. However, sorting through the myriad of medical research articles requires the latest in computer equipment and skills. Thus, evidence-based techniques are more difficult for physicians to access in areas with limited resources. Furthermore, critics espouse that evidence-based medicine compromises the 'art of medicine' by taking away the physicians ability to treat patients on an individual basis (Zuger, 1997). <!-- margin note: evidence-based medicine -->

Another important component in the future of health care for many of our nation's citizens is **Telemedicine**. Telemedicine is defined as a system that electronically transports a consulting physician's expertise to a site at a distant facility where it is needed. It can be as complex as multipoint videoconferencing with high-resolution image transfer or as simple as faxing a copy of a radiograph to a consulting physician (Institute of Medicine, 1996). <!-- margin note: Telemedicine -->

The most common clinical uses for telemedicine are diagnostic consults, medical data transmissions, and management of chronic illnesses. By the end of 1997, nearly 30% of rural hospitals in the U.S. used telemedicine to deliver patient care and over 35 federal organizations, 10 state governments, and numerous private organizations sponsored initiatives in over 40 states. Already 15 states offer some telemedicine coverage under their Medicaid programs and California and Louisiana have enacted legislation mandating coverage under their private insurance plans for telemedicine consultation services. The financial bottom line of telemedicine in America is that approximately $200 million can be saved annually by its implementation.

Summary and Conclusions

This chapter reviewed the components of a managed care system. These involve: contracted provider networks with primary care and specialty providers; patient access systems to clinicians; utilization management/case management with practice guidelines; claims payment/fiscal controls including capitation; customer service as it relates to both patient and provider; and quality management activities and programs. This chapter also presented future directions in health care delivery and discussed the increasing prevalence of capitation and its impact on providers as an important issue to be dealt with in the ethics of quality care. Finally, this chapter presented the concepts of disease-state management and evidence-based medicine, and introduced the advanced technology of telemedicine with its implications for cost savings in the delivery of services to underserved populations.

The various health problems of the fictional Symington family will now be presented. The authors encourage the reader to problem-solve the most effective treatment in a managed care setting for an adolescent's asthma attack, a breast cancer diagnosis and an adult's back problems. Based on information presented in this chapter, the authors propose solutions to these treatments at the end of each case study.

The Symington Case Continued

Problem #1: Ricky has an asthma attack

Although the Symingtons have just enrolled in an HMO, Ricky is still not taking all of his prescribed asthma medication. While raking leaves in his back yard, Ricky becomes dyspneic. He tries to self-medicate with his bronchodialator, which has gone past its expiration date, but his condition worsens. As his former physician used to hospitalize him for similar symptoms, Kathy packs Ricky an overnight bag and drives to the nearest hospital in the late afternoon expecting him to spend the night in the hospital.

The emergency room physician evaluates Ricky and determines that he has an acute exacerbation of his asthma with moderate shortness of breath, mildly hypoxemic, but a normal chest X-ray. The ER physician begins initial treatment with a bolus of intravenous (IV) steroids and nebulized albuterol. Since the hospital is not part of the Symingtons HMO plan, the ER physician contacts his primary care physician. The ER Physician recommends that Ricky be admitted overnight to stabilize his condition. What should Ricky's primary care physician do? His options include the following:

1. Admit Ricky and see him immediately.
2. Admit Ricky and see him the next day.
3. Transfer Ricky to a network hospital.
4. Have Ricky remain in the ER and check on his status in an hour.
5. Visit Ricky in the ER to evaluate his condition.

A Proposed Solution to Problem #1

Dr. Brown, Ricky's primary care physician, calls the ER physician back in an hour to check on Ricky's condition. The ER physician tells Dr. Brown that Ricky is experiencing no shortness of breath and only mild wheezing. After reviewing his peak flow and ABGs, Dr. Brown instructs the ER physician to disconnect Ricky's IV and indicates that he can go home. However, Ricky is to start on new medications that evening which his family can now afford with the low co-pay. Ricky must be seen in Dr. Brown's office the next morning.

Ricky arrives at Dr. Brown's office feeling much better. Dr. Brown determines that Ricky's peak flow and pulse oximetry is satisfactory and that he has only mild wheezing. Dr. Brown suggests that Ricky needs guidance in learning how to control his asthma and refers him to Ms. Smith, a nurse in his office who has been trained in the 'best practices' of asthma management by the Symington's HMO plan. Initially, Ms. Smith, teaches Ricky how to monitor his peak flow and to self-medicate. She also tells his parents the procedures they need to follow at their HMO when Ricky's asthma can no longer be self-managed. Ms. Smith sees Ricky on two more occasions during the next few weeks to monitor his condition and to make sure that he has mastered self-management. During this time Ms. Smith also consults with Dr. Brown to keep him up-to-date on Ricky's progress. Dr. Brown sees Ricky a month later and concurs with the asthma management plan that Ms. Smith has set up for Ricky. Follow-up visits with Ms. Smith are scheduled as needed.

This proposal is an excellent example of how an HMO can effectively manage a chronic condition such as asthma. The HMO was able to improve the quality of care and at the same time reduce costs. For example, HMO data revealed that there was a high prevalence of bronchial asthma within its population that was not being adequately controlled. **Underutilization** of inhaled steroids and inattention to environmental triggers resulted in a significant use of ER and inpatient facilities. After training its health care providers in 'best practices' of asthma management, the HMO was able to eliminate the high costs of treatment by redesigning the asthma care process and initiating patient education programs.

Problem #2: Kathy Develops Breast Cancer

Kathy was diagnosed two years ago with lobular carcinoma *in situ* and treated by Dr. Jones, a breast surgeon specialist in the Midwest where she had been living. Kathy's pre-malignant condition is a marker for possible breast cancer, but if it is identified early, is fully treatable. Just before Kathy moved to the East, she had a mammogram and follow-up consultation with Dr. Jones. Dr. Jones told Kathy that she wanted to review her mammogram with the Radiologist and would recommend Dr. Adams, a colleague in the East, if further follow-up was needed. After consulting with the Radiologist, Dr. Jones realized that Kathy needed a repeat mammogram with magnification, contacted Dr. Adams with this information and sent him all Kathy's records and test results. Dr. Adams did not notify Kathy.

Kathy contacts her new HMO to determine if she can see Dr. Adams. The HMO indicates that they will not cover the costs of her being treated by Dr. Adams because he is not a network provider. The HMO clerk telephones Kathy to say that before a specialist can see her in her health care plan she first needs to be seen by a primary care physician. At this time Kathy is unaware that she needs a new mammogram. Preoccupied with the tasks of settling into a new community, she waits to schedule a visit with a primary care physician because she is frustrated with the process. Several months later Kathy visits Dr. Brown, her new primary care physician. Dr. Brown then contacts Dr. Adams to whom her medical records had been sent.

Dr. Brown recognizes the concern expressed by Dr. Jones six months earlier regarding a follow-up mammogram with magnification. He immediately arranges for Kathy to have another mammogram. Her test results reveal that she has an aggressive breast cancer tumor that is estrogen receptor negative. Kathy is stunned by this diagnosis, as she was unaware that questions had arisen pertaining to her mammogram six months ago. Dr. Brown refers Kathy to a breast surgeon in the HMO who begins an appropriate treatment regimen. While Kathy's breast cancer was caught at an early stage, how could it have been detected much earlier?

A Proposed Solution to Problem #2

Kathy's case is an example of what happens when a patient gets lost in the system. Her records did not get transferred properly from the Midwest to the East because there was a lack of communication between health care providers and patient. Even though Dr. Jones referred Kathy to a colleague in the East she should have informed Kathy that she needed a new mammogram. Should Dr. Adams have followed up with Kathy regarding Dr. Jones' concerns even if he never saw her? There may be a fracturing of the original patient-doctor relationship when a patient moves to another city.

On the other hand, Kathy became frustrated with the rules of the HMO when the system would not budge to let her see the breast surgeon specialist her former doctor had recommended. This type of frustration abetted her 'denial' and fostered non-compliance with appropriate follow-up care. Instead of becoming frustrated with having to see a primary care physician first, which resulted in a delayed diagnosis of breast cancer, Kathy needed to understand how the plan her family selected worked. It is important that patients and providers understand the parameters and rules of a given managed care system.

Problem #3: Michael develops severe back problems

While Michael was moving heavy boxes in the basement to help his daughter Renee locate some of her books packed away from their move, he experienced severe pain in his lower back. Since it was late afternoon, Michael telephoned his primary care physician, Dr. Brown, and was told by the nurse that he could be seen the next morning. In the meantime, Michael was instructed to take over-the-counter pain medication, apply heat to his back and rest. Michael went to bed early that evening, had a restless night and woke up the next morning with increased pain.

Dr. Brown examines Michael the next morning and suspects that he has a ruptured disk and will probably need surgery. He prescribes Motrin, Valium and bedrest and refers Michael to Dr. Green, a neurosurgeon in the HMO network. Michael calls Dr. Green and to his dismay he cannot see him for 10 days. Michael is concerned about the time he is missing from work since his pain is so intense that he is unable to perform his duties.

Michael is finally seen by Dr. Green and describes his symptoms. Dr. Green notes that Michael has pain in his mid lumbosacral (LS) area, extending to the right buttock and posterior thigh above the level of his knee. Also, Dr. Green determines that Michael has decreased right ankle reflex, slight weakness, dorsiflexion of the right great toe, and equivocal right straight-leg raising test. Dr. Green prescribes a MRI of Michael's LS spine and tells him to continue taking Motrin and rest as much as possible. Michael returns to work per Dr. Green's recommendation, however he is significantly restricted in the duties he can perform.

When Dr. Green receives the MRI results, his office telephones Michael to set up another appointment. Michael's symptoms have improved since he last saw Dr. Green but he is still experiencing pain. The MRI reveals 'anterior bulge, disc at L3–L4, without definite herniation and Grade II spondylolisthesis L4–L5'. Dr. Green recommends a lumbar laminectomy, a surgical procedure to correct Michael's back pain problem. However, Dr. Green must obtain authorization from the HMO to perform this surgery, and instructs his staff to begin this process. Michael is impatient and asks Dr. Green why he has to wait for authorization before he has the surgery. Dr. Green explains that he could be severely penalized if he failed to obtain prior authorization.

The authorization process includes the following steps:
1. Dr. Green fills out a standard form documenting Michael's case and sends this to the HMO's nurse reviewer.
2. The nurse reviewer inputs this data into their information system.
3. Michael is contacted by the nurse reviewer and answers a series of standard questions which are then entered into the information system.
4. The nurse reviewer then utilizes the decision matrix data from the HMO's information system and determines that the proposed surgical procedure 'fails appropriateness **criteria**'.
5. The nurse reviewer sends the input and output data from the decision matrix to the HMO's Associate Medical Director.
6. The Associate Medical Director reviews the hard copy of the case, and contacts Dr. Green to discuss the facts of the case and the treatment plan for Michael.

7. The Associate Medical Director does not overrule the initial HMO's denial of surgery because there is insufficient neurologic findings indicating a herniated disc and insufficient trial of non-operative therapy. The Associate Medical Director contacts Dr. Green to let him know they denied the surgical procedure. He is told that he can appeal this case for a final ruling. What is Dr. Green to do?

A Proposed Solution to Problem #3

Dr. Green decides not to appeal the denial and instead pursues a course of non-operative treatment for Michael. He consults with Dr. Brown, Michael's primary care physician, regarding a new treatment plan. Drs. Green and Brown concur that Michael should attend 'Back School' that is offered by a physical therapy department in the HMO's network. Michael is also to continue with Motrin and restrict lifting activities both at work and at home.

While Michael is disappointed that he cannot have the lumbar laminectomy, he agrees to the treatment plan proposed by his primary care physician in consultation with his neurosurgeon. Michael is to follow-up with Dr. Brown in a month.

Michael begins an eight week program of 'Back School' which he attends twice a week. The rehabilitation process includes modalities such as heat and ultra-sound, manipulation through myofascial release, weight loss, and a home exercise program. The use of medications is limited to anti-inflammatory agents. Michael is compliant with the program and returns to see Dr. Brown with significantly decreased pain. Dr. Green is pleased with Michael's progress. Michael graduates from 'Back School' the following month with no pain and therefore functioning normally. Michael's only restriction is to avoid heavy lifting. Letters from the physical therapy department are sent to Dr. Brown stating Michael's success with the 'Back School.'

5. Disease Prevention and Health Promotion

While managed care is often perceived as focusing primarily on managing cost, quality, and access to health care, it has as an inherent principle the management of an enrolled population's health. This involves the one-on-one patient-provider encounter as well as **population-based strategies** to promote the overall health of their enrollees. Although managed care plans see these population-based strategies of health promotion and disease prevention as their ultimate goals, only the more mature plans evolved to this ideal.

Many plans are extending preventive services to the broader community as they realize that promoting the health of the community is integral to the health of their enrollees. Therefore, physicians and allied health care professionals will have to learn non-office based approaches to complement their patient-centered care if they are to treat their populations effectively. This approach requires gathering information about the community that they serve (i.e., its demographics, sociocultural beliefs and practices), and the **epidemiology** of health problems prevalent in the community. Thus, the managed care field must pay considerable attention to the development and application of the basic concepts of public health and prevention.

Among the greatest achievements in modern medicine's effort to reduce human suffering was the development of prevention techniques, such as the Salk polio vaccine, that allow the health care system to eliminate the emergence of disease as opposed to focusing on the treatment of individual cases once they occur. While achievements as dramatic as those made by the Salk vaccine are not a daily occur-

epidemiology

rence, practitioners in the managed care field are increasingly cognizant of the importance of prevention in disease control.

Some examples of preventive population-based strategies that managed care plans might adopt to promote health involve monitoring the proportion of female enrollees who had annual pap smears, or the proportion of pregnant women who had pre-natal care. Other preventive interventions could include sending enrollees announcements to remind parents about childhood vaccinations, free blood pressure and cholesterol screenings, and group counseling sessions dealing with weight reduction, smoking cessation or stress management.

Levels of Prevention

disease prevention

prevalence

incidence

When speaking of the **prevention** of disease there are two approaches on which to focus. The first emphasizes a reduction in the number of people who already have a disorder, or the prevalence of the disorder. The second approach emphasizes reductions in the number of people who develop the disorder anew, reducing the incidence of the disorder. These two concepts, prevalence and incidence, are the main factors that the health professions use to distinguish among the three levels of prevention. These three levels are as follows: tertiary, secondary and primary prevention (Caplan, 1964).

tertiary prevention

Tertiary prevention involves the reduction of the prevalence of a disorder in a given population. It is often confused with rehabilitation, which focuses on reducing the severity of a disorder in an individual rather than in a population. In contrast, tertiary prevention means that the focus of intervention is on a population of disordered individuals. For example, policies that encourage work with autistic children in their home school systems rather than in residential facilities would constitute tertiary preventive interventions. Keeping children in their communities reduces the chances that a long period of removal will make integration into the community problematic, thus exacerbating the deleterious affects of the disorder itself. Not only does this approach better address the needs of the patient, but it is also cost-effective.

It is paradoxical that tertiary prevention, intent upon reducing the prevalence of disease, may actually do the opposite. This occurs when intervention into severe and intractable illnesses prolongs life by increasing individual's adaptive skills without actually ridding them of their original health problem. The next level of prevention, secondary prevention, speaks to this paradox by finding and intervening earlier, thus increasing the chances that significant numbers will be able to return to the ranks of the healthy.

Secondary prevention is intervention early in the disease process. In order for secondary prevention to avoid the paradox of increased prevalence of disorders often found with tertiary preventive interventions, it is necessary that early identification or detection be followed by effective intervention. The third and final level of prevention is primary prevention that does not focus on prevalence at all. Its target is the rate at which new cases of an illness are identified. Primary prevention is closest to what layperson's mean when they discuss preventing something, although arriving at a definitive meaning requires consideration of diverse opinions from multiple disciplines. For example, interventions with adolescent cancer patients that reduce the incidence of depression among them would be primary prevention in that being a cancer patient is neither necessary nor sufficient for the development of depression. *secondary prevention* *primary prevention*

Strategies of Disease Prevention

Like public health's concept of prevention, managed care's goal is to control physical diseases and focus on decreasing the rate of occurrence of diseases in a population or a whole community rather than on curing diseases once they have begun. In prevention terms, disease can be interrupted in four ways: 1. strengthen the person who may get the disease (host inoculation); 2. remove the cause of the disease (the pathological agent); 3. remove the mechanisms by which the disease is spread; and 4. change the environment to reduce the chances that host and pathological agent come together (Bloom, 1985).

When the managed care environment adopts prevention, particularly primary prevention, it has the potential to interrupt the course of disease in multiple ways. These include interventions focused on the host, the pathological agent (i.e., stress), or the environment (i.e., social support for stress). The American Public Health Association identified six categories of preventable diseases, all of known etiology. Prevention of these diseases illustrates the mix of host inoculation, environmental manipulation, and control of the disease that may be required to mount effective primary prevention programs (Bloom, 1985).

Poisoning causes the first group of preventable diseases. Poisons may be intentionally or accidentally ingested in many forms, includ- *poisoning*

---

ing drugs, solvents, and industrial toxins, and can lead to chronic brain syndromes. One prevention strategy requires that the host's lifestyle be altered in order to avoid the poisoning agent. Another preventive strategy is to change the environment to reduce the chances that host and pathological agent make contact. Managed care organizations can accomplish this through parent education programs that emphasize the importance of making the poisoning agents unavailable. For instance, removing lead paint from windowsills so that children cannot ingest the lead so readily is an example of altering the environment to prevent poisoning.

infections

Diseases caused by infections such as rubella and syphilis during the fetal period, or measles and influenza during childhood, are in a second category of preventable brain damage. The managed care environment can prevent these diseases through strengthening the host (the child) with inoculations, or by treating the mother for fetally transmitted diseases, thus removing the pathological agent.

genetic disorder

Genetic disorders comprise the third category of preventable diseases. Special diets during infancy can prevent diseases such as phenylketonuria, preventing the retardation that would otherwise result. Genetic counseling can also reduce the incidence of genetic disorders.

nutritional deficiency

The fourth category of preventable diseases is those resulting from nutritional deficiency, such as pellagra and beriberi, which increase the chance of mental retardation and other cognitive and perceptual disorders. Host inoculation in the form of nutritional supplements in the diet can prevent these disorders.

accidental or intentional injuries

Disorders caused by injuries, accidental or intentional, to the nervous system comprise the fifth category of preventable health problems. These can be prevented by inoculating the host with such things as motorcycle helmets, removing the pathological agent by making handguns less readily available, and changing the environment through mechanisms such as safe speed limits.

systemic disorders

The final category of preventable diseases consists of general systemic disorders such as toxemia of pregnancy and prematurity. Educating pregnant women concerning the importance of prenatal care in order to enhance the fetal environment can prevent the negative consequences of these health problems for newborns.

The above discussion of the six categories of disorders of known etiology provides examples of the categorization of preventive interventions. Since managed care organizations are responsible for the health of large populations, they can have a significant impact on interrupting these preventable health problems.

Health Promotion

Health promotion can occur in the absence of a disease of known etiology, and consists of interventions that have a positive but non-specific effect on health. Provided to individuals, groups or even large populations, its focus is on the enhancement of well-being rather than illness. For example, mental health promotion might include cognitive and behavioral interventions such as those to reduce anger, regulate anxiety and increase positive cognition in order to enhance personal harmony and well-being. Mental health promotion programs are burgeoning, and can be found in schools, health service organizations, businesses, industries and municipal governments (Mrazek and Haggerty, 1994). On the personal level, meditation, massage, yoga and acupuncture are all being used to promote health and well-being. The economic costs and benefits of mental health promotion are hard to define in conventional terms, but these efforts are becoming quite substantial in both the public and private sectors as well as in the managed care field. Managed care organizations cannot ignore these health promotion pursuits in regard to their enrolled populations, as the cost-effectiveness of these programs could be substantial in the long run.

enhancement of well-being

Health Protection

Finally, health protection is a public health mechanism that seeks to reduce the number of health hazards in the environment through the use of public regulatory activities. An example of such a regulatory activity would be controlling the availability of drugs and alcoholic beverages or regulating occupational safety activities (Pew, 1995). Also, it is found that good schools can have a profound protective effect on students at the secondary level as the schools reinforce good work and behavior, avail teachers to deal with problems and accord responsibility to students (Mrazek and Haggerty, 1994).

reduce health hazards

Identifying Target Populations

Prevention programs adopted by managed care organizations and administered to groups of people are identified in several ways. Bloom (1985) describes prevention programs as community wide, milestone or high-risk programs.

In a **communitywide program**, all of the people in a given geographic area receive the intervention. In the **milestone approach**, every individual in a population who reaches a certain hurdle is a member of the target group. The milestones are usually thought of as critical life transitions, such as being fired, becoming a parent for the first time, or going away to college. Programs include efforts such as outplacement counseling for fired employees and orientation programs for entering college students. High-risk programs focus on populations rather than on events. For example, children of alcoholics, adults with chronic illnesses, and teenage mothers are all groups who are vulnerable. Managed care organizations can institute programs that reduce the chances that members of these high-risk groups manifest a disorder (Rickel and Becker, 1998).

No single method for identifying recipients of preventive interventions is clearly superior to all the rest. Communitywide and milestone programs are often expensive because many of the people who get the program will not need it. As is true with the distribution of other resources in our society, those most likely to avail themselves of milestone or communitywide interventions are those least in need. There are also critical flaws in the **high-risk approach** to identifying clients of prevention programs. Individuals who are at risk are usually overidentified in terms of the number who would actually develop a problem without preventive intervention. This labeling can actually increase the risk to an individual, as its effects can be profoundly disturbing (Hobbs, 1975).

The most cost-effective method for identifying client populations in terms of optimized gain and minimized risk is probably a combination of the labeling approach with one of the 'take all comers' approaches. Establishing a milestone program for those entering high school, and then further screening entrants using one or more risk indices is an example of such an approach. The use of multiple risk bases in an already selected population of needy individuals decreases the chances of labeling children unnecessarily. The reduction of the milestone population through the use of person-centered risk bases decreases the numbers who receive intervention, and therefore the cost.

Risk Analysis

Epidemiology, a subspecialty within public health, determines who becomes ill, how many people have a given illness, why people become ill, and what can be done to stop them from becoming ill. Risk is a key concept in epidemiology because determining who is at risk for illness becomes a wedge in tracking and preventing illnesses more efficiently. For managed care organizations, identifying risk factors allows for the most efficient use of program resources in that programs can recruit individuals most in need of an intervention (Hough, 1985).

Risk factors are usually in one of two categories, depending on when they occur relative to the onset of symptoms. The first group, predisposing factors, are those that occur several months to years prior to the onset of symptoms. These can be further subdivided into those that can be modified and those that are, by their very nature, unmodifiable. Unmodifiable or unavoidable risk factors include such demographics as gender, social class, age and ethnicity. For example, women may be more prone to depression than men, adolescents may be more prone to pathological reactions to loneliness than members of any other age group, and the offspring of schizophrenics may be more at risk for the development of psychotic symptoms themselves.

There are two implications for prevention to consider with unmodifiable risk factors. The first is that early intervention is critical for offsetting the vulnerability created by the presence of these factors. The second is that these unmodifiable predisposing factors may increase in power by societal reaction to people who carry them. The stigma of being a minority group member, a girl, or the child of a schizophrenic may increase the chances that a disorder will become manifest.

The second group of predisposing risk factors is called modifiable, or avoidable, risk factors. These are all events that occur early in life that increases the chances for later disorder. For example, early interventions, such as home environment and personality, can alter developing a disorder later on in life. Programs that involve children with low self-esteem can increase their self-esteem and render them more resilient in the face of stressors. Another group of modifiable risk factors includes demographic variables (i.e., education, occupation, income and marital status). Microlevel interventions can alter these modifiable risk factors as well. Seeking to change an individual's occupation to a higher status group with greater access to resources for dealing with stressors can blunt these factors directly.

In contrast to predisposing factors, which occur much earlier than the onset of the symptoms, precipitating factors occur just before the

---

onset of symptoms and indeed trigger this onset. Investigation into the role of life events as precipitants of disorder accelerated appreciation of the significance of life events. Researchers are also actively investigating life strain, daily stress and macro-environmental traumas as precipitating factors in illness (Dohrenwend et al., 1979).

The literature on life events consistently indicates that some events, whether singly or in close temporal proximity with other events, places individuals at considerable risk. Documented stressors include events such as divorce in the family, bereavement, or immigration. The implications of research on life events for the design of prevention programs are several (Hough, 1985). Populations can be taught to anticipate stress in order to avoid becoming overwhelmed. Second, by increasing a population's resilience, the level of social competence in them can increase. Children starting junior high school, for instance, can be taught survival skills beforehand that will reduce the degree to which the school transition is a risk factor. Third, interventions can be designed to help individuals in at-risk populations to alter their perceptions of risk factors and lower their estimations of the possible stressful impact of events. Fourth, programs designed for at-risk groups, such as newly divorce or newly bereaved people, can teach specific coping techniques. To address the needs of such populations, event centered support groups evolved and incorporated into community practice.

Summary and Conclusions

The ultimate goal and hallmark of managed care is to promote self-care and wellness among patients. As mentioned, preventive programs instituted by managed care organizations are routine physical examinations and health assessments, immunizations, mammograms, PAP tests, and prenatal care visits. This chapter presented the three levels of prevention: primary, secondary and tertiary; as well as strategies of disease prevention, health protection and health promotion. Suggested programs to discourage unhealthy behaviors and lower the risk of ill health include smoking cessation, stress reduction and nutritional intervention. Also, this chapter outlined the identification of target populations and discussed risk assessment. Increasingly, there are positive outcomes associated with prevention programs, but more long-term study is needed to determine the benefits of managed care organizations' prevention programs.

6. New Challenges and Opportunities

Currently, the membership in HMOs exceeds 50 million individuals – a number which may more than double in the next five years. With this rapid growth of managed care, have come major changes in the health care system. Witness the increase in the for-profit hospital chains and the decrease in the non-profit hospitals, especially in rural and low-income urban areas. The delivery of health care continues to be divided up by various commercial enterprises – pharmaceutical benefits companies, home health care groups, mental health carve-outs, physical medicine and rehabilitation groups, to name just a few. It is safe to say that the United States has not seen a massive political, economic, and social movement on the scale of managed care since the era of civil rights.

Managed care is here to stay, at least as the U.S. enters the 21st century. However, patients and providers are calling for reform in many areas. Therefore, it becomes vital to elaborate on several key issues relevant to the future existence of this form of health care. This chapter explores in depth a few of the challenges and opportunities facing the managed care industry.

One of the most important issues requiring attention is the ethical basis of managed care. The halls of academia are debating this issue, and therefore it must be brought to the forefront so that all interested parties can take part in this serious discussion. This chapter enumerates on the 'adversarial vs. collegial' relationship between patients, providers and the managed care organizations as a surgence in lawsuits and negative press continue to bombard the managed care industry. Also discussed is the move from extensive reporting to targeted reporting by providers. The concept of quality control, an essential component of managed care, is presented in the context of the standardization of reporting systems as well as in the area of accreditation. Finally, this chapter examines the management styles of managed care organizations, both micromanagement and macromanagement, as this is one area in which legislative reform is concentrating.

Ethics and Managed Care

The expansion of managed care in the U.S. marketplace raised important ethical issues for virtually everyone involved in the process: health care providers, corporate providers of health benefits, consumers, policy planners and managed care firms. For the most part, the ethical issues that arise in managed care involve the relationship between costs of health care services, the quality of health care and access to health care.

The ethical basis of managed care is not widely understood. Many clinicians propose that it is sometimes used to achieve rapid savings. These opponents contend that when oversight and controls on expenditures increase, quality of care will inversely decrease. However, proponents of managed care argue that quality is not compromised, but is equal to or better than unmanaged care. Furthermore, managed care seeks to produce the maximum value for an enrolled population from the limited resources available. These opposing viewpoints of managed care are an integral basis for a discussion of ethics.

Using the American Medical Association's Principles of Medical Ethics as a basis, Sabin (1996) proposes four additional ethical principles for clinicians practicing in managed care settings. These four principles involve: 1. Clinicians need to care for their patients in a patient-centered relationship as well as serve as a protector of society's resources; 2. Clinicians need to recommend the most economical patient treatment unless there is evidence that a more expensive treatment would produce a better outcome; 3. Clinicians need to advocate for justice in the health care system; and 4. Clinicians need to determine what type of health care is delivered based on standards determined by the population and agreed upon by the patient.

With regard to Principle 1, the clinician has the dual responsibility of serving as an advocate for their patient while at the same time serving as an advocate for the health plans' population or the larger community. For example, physicians face a responsibility toward patients whose needs are sometimes in direct economic conflict with managed care systems. These patients include the poor, the chronically mentally ill, or the terminally ill who are frequently unable to advocate for their own interests. Rather than passively follow practice guidelines, the clinician has to advocate for the care of these patients. At the same time, the clinician needs to consider the costs of allocating valuable resources to promote health and prevent illness in the population served. Thus, it is vital that clinicians communicate their dual roles to individual patients and the populations they serve. patient vs. community advocacy

In Principle 2, the clinician should recommend the most appropriate and least expensive treatment unless there is significant evidence that a more costly alternative treatment is superior. In this way, clinicians can manage costs more effectively and use their time efficiently in order to achieve wider access and benefits for their enrolled population. While many clinicians and consumers in the U.S. do not agree with this approach to practice, it is the ethical foundation for health care in the United Kingdom and Canada. In these countries, patients give their providers 'informed consent' in that they want to promote the greatest good for the greatest number of citizens and are willing to levy taxes on themselves to support the entire population's health care. promote greatest good for greatest number

Principle 3 states that ethical clinicians in their stewardship role need to advocate for justice in the health care system, as well as for the welfare of their patients. The concept of justice used here includes three major dimensions. The first dimension encompasses the fact that providers as well as the public should demand that managed care produce the best results with the available resources for the involved population. The second dimension states that providers and the public insist on a health care system of informed consent whereby medical choices are made by participants with the full understanding of the consequences (i.e. access, cost, etc.). Finally, providers and the public cannot allow for discrimination of health resources to occur. Patients should not be denied access to an adequate standard of health care because of ethnic origin, race, creed, socioeconomic status, age, sex, or sexual orientation. advocate for justice

Lastly, Principle 4 deals with rationing as it occurs in the course of establishing what type of health care is to be delivered. Both the affected health population and the individual patient need to agree rationing of health care

---

upon the rationing. Sabin provides examples of four different ways in which the inevitable rationing can occur. The first exemplifies the U.S. health care system, where uninsurance and underinsurance achieve the necessitated rationing. Sabin regards this form of rationing as unethical. The second example of rationing occurs when insurance companies put a 'cap' on medical services provided and constrain the type and amount of health care provided. Thus, patients who require treatment beyond the allowable cap are being rationed. The third example achieves rationing by prioritizing medical treatment, as in Oregon where the legislature allocates a specific amount of money to health care based on a prioritized list of medical services and will not pay for treatment beyond an established point. For this type of rationing to work, it is important that the affected population understands the prioritized list. Finally, determining what is 'medically necessary' is another way to achieve rationing. However, a quagmire of moral reasoning surrounds the concept of **medical necessity**. Who determines what is medically necessary? How does one determine what is medically necessary? In the U.S., the courts are the final arbiters but their decisions are significantly being influenced by the changing terms of health insurance policies, by utilization review agreements, by the quality of medical evidence and by evolving community standards.

medical necessity

This overview of the ethical foundations of managed care will better prepare health care providers for the difficult resource allocation decisions they will be asked to make. This chapter furthers the discussion on additional challenges facing clinicians in a managed care environment, as the political and ethical debate about medical choices and trade-offs only continues to gather steam.

Adversarial vs. Collegial

Just as with other movements for the general welfare, there are growing adversarial relationships between forces active in the delivery of managed care. The tensions inherent in any change gave birth and nourishment to a backlash against managed care organizations. On the legislative side, 1996 saw 35 states enact 56 laws aimed at the regulation of services provided by managed care organizations. Eighteen states passed laws prohibiting clauses in physician contracts forbidding the disclosure of monetary bonuses and/or discussion of treatment options not paid for by the managed care physicians from being dismissed 'without just cause'. Termination of a contract 'without just cause' usually resulted from economical reasons, rarely from competency issues.

Approximately one quarter of the states have legislation requiring managed care organizations to pay for hospital emergency room visits according to a 'prudent layperson's' concept of an emergent situation. This is any condition that a layman reasonably fears might result in significant morbidity and/or mortality. Prior to this legislation, many managed care organizations refused payment for emergency room visits not deemed emergencies by various criteria. By far, the most visible legislation concerns restrictions placed by managed care organizations on the coverage of the number of post partum inpatient days following an uncomplicated delivery. Almost half of the states now have laws requiring managed care organizations to provide hospital coverage for at least 48 hours after delivery.

Access to physicians and allied health care professionals other than primary care doctors is a major issue in the backlash against managed care organizations. The state of Kentucky enacted legislation that requires HMOs to provide direct access to chiropractors. In New York, HMOs must allow women two check-ups per year by their obstetrician-gynecologist without referral from a primary care physician. Several other states, including Alabama, Colorado, Connecticut, Indiana, Maine, Maryland, Oregon, Utah and Virginia, have similar laws concerning access to obstetric/gynecologic physicians. As the use of alternative therapies (homeopathic, acupuncture, herbal, etc.) increases in popularity, these practitioners will also demand legislation in order to receive financial coverage for and access to their services from the managed care organizations.

While the amount of legislation regulating managed care organizations continues to grow, so also is the amount of lawsuits hitting the managed care organizations – many of them high profile with large financial settlements. The majority of the suits deal with the issues of access to care, especially experimental treatment and delay of care. Experimental treatment is hard to define, in broadest terms it is care that is new and not widely accepted due to lack of proven efficacy. In many cases, the local standard of care plays a major role in defining what is experimental. Recently, the definition of experimental treatment was challenged in the case of bone marrow transplants for women with advanced or treatment-resistant breast carcinoma. Frequently, the managed care organizations denied coverage for this procedure, noting lack of outcome-based research demonstrating a clear survival benefit. Conflict arises between a medical culture that grew accustomed to few restraints (especially financial) on experimentation and a managed care culture whose foundation rests on financial conservatism. Added to this explosive mixture is a patient population accustomed to the latest medical technologies and treatment modalities.

With the 'gatekeeper' model of managed care, many argue that there are delays in patients receiving specialist care. By its very nature, specialty care tends to be expensive; thus, a hallmark of managed care is the close regulation of membership access to this care. High profile suits with much media attention focused on patients who suffered severe morbidity or even mortality due to delays in receiving specialist attention and/or various diagnostic work-ups.

The relationship between physicians and managed care organizations provided much fuel for the recent backlash against managed care organizations. The tremendous growth in managed care in the last ten years left many physicians uncertain of the future. In particular, physicians witnessed the lessening of their control over medical management. In response, physicians are forming novel organizations to increase their bargaining power. In December of 1996, a group of physicians in Tucson, Arizona joined the Federation of Physicians and Dentists – marking the first time physicians employed by a for-profit managed care organization unionized in the United States. In New York, doctors established both a union representing physicians employed by the public hospitals, as well as the Union of American Physicians and Dentists representing the interests of physicians employed in government and university settings.

In addition to unions, physicians merged into large groups of both primary care and specialty care. These groups, such as Med-Partners and Caremark, successfully competed against large managed care organizations for the right to offer health plans directly to employers. Physician groups also banded/together to increase direct bargaining power with the managed care organization. For example, Primary Care LCC based in Boston, successfully negotiated a contract with a Massachusetts managed care organization to provide care to some of its 40,000 members. Physician–hospital organizations also formed to provide closer co-operation between large hospitals (especially academic centers) and their medical staffs. While still in their infancy, the physician–hospital organizations hope to increase their bargaining with local managed care organizations by merging their services.

Whereas the difficulties that physicians experienced with managed care organizations reduced their autonomy in regard to patient care, the relationships among physicians is also eroding this autonomy. Documented rifts between primary care physicians and specialists lead to wars with few winners. It is true that specialists who have longer training command greater reimbursement from the managed care organizations. However, primary care physicians need to recognize this advantage and work to have this reimbursement gap reduced (Shenkin, 1995).

While the adversarial situations are easy to pinpoint (especially with the growing media attentions), the collegial aspects are often more difficult to define. The growth of managed care increased the interest in outcome research and thus provided the incentive for development of various large databases. This enabled physicians and researchers to gain rapid access to large amounts of demographic and clinical data. Managed care also served to broaden the concept of outcome to include more patient focused outcomes, including satisfaction and quality of life. Most managed care organizations actively seek input from the membership, through various methods like questionnaires and verbal interviews. In addition, many managed care organizations also have as part of their corporate structure membership panels that serve to advise them on various consumer issues.

Managed care organizations are also beginning to form collegial partnerships with academic health care centers in order to provide education for both students and residents. Clearly, it is in the best interest of managed care organizations to support medical education due to the gain in early exposure of new physicians and trainees to the managed care philosophy. These physicians will have a clearer understanding of the principals of medical care delivery under managed care and will be better equipped to function within the culture of the managed care organization. Providing educational opportunities also helps the managed care organization to foster a collegial working relationship with both the local and the national medical educational communities. Providing educational support affords the managed care organization a certain amount of prestige among the local patient population.

In the past, the medical community often viewed the regional academic medical center as the authority on medical conditions, especially the difficult to diagnose and the difficult to treat. As managed care organizations become associated with academic medical centers and training, they will enjoy a certain portion of the prestige. What remains to be fully delineated are the care concepts and competencies that should be gained by both students and resident physicians training in a managed care organization setting. Clearly, the managed care organization atmosphere can provide additional emphasis in such topics as resource allocation, team health care management, health care financing, health promotion, and risk management. Finally, how education will differ between the for-profit and non-profit managed care organization settings remains unresolved.

How managed care organizations contribute to the funding of medical research continues to be a major stumbling block in the mergers of academic medical centers and these organizations. For years, hospital revenue, clinical practice revenue, and departmental moneys funded and subsidized research. In 1993, approximately $816 million went towards research in a medical school, about $0.10 of every faculty practice plan dollar collected (Moy et al., 1997). As for-profit organizations purchase academic medical centers, it is clear that they must closely observe expenditures for research.

Currently, many hospital-based academic physicians may see their funding for research activities lessen as clinical revenues decrease due to reductions in physician reimbursements. Without clear extramural support, many research physicians are being forced to increase their clinical activities in order to maintain financial support for their research endeavors. It is well known that managed care plans tend to select physicians and hospitals on the basis of cost. Thus, support of research can erode as market competition increases and as a result, medical schools depend more on clinical revenues. So, departments in more competitive settings may encourage greater patient care activities, at the sacrifice of their research and teaching activities.

An interesting study published in the *Journal of the American Medical Association* in the July 16, 1997 issue, looked at the relationship between market competition and the activities and attitudes of medical school faculty. Preliminary findings suggest that the competitiveness of local markets directly impact faculty research, clinical activities and perceptions of departmental climate (Campbell et al., 1997). The study found that i, the rate of publication for clinical researchers has decreased in the past three years in competitive markets, ii, the percentage of young faculty with patient care responsibilities was greater in the competitive markets and iii, the faculty perceived lower levels of departmental community and co-operation in the most competitive markets.

There are several possible explanations for these results. One theory is that in the more competitive markets, academic health centers may be unable to support clinical researchers with revenues they receive from patient care. Another theory suggests that in the more competitive markets the volume of clinical research performed in academic health centers may be lower as a result of a greater presence of private, for-profit contract research organizations. Strategies to protect clinical research missions need to focus on academic health centers in competitive markets. Solutions include: channel more of the institutional funds to faculty who conduct clinical research, increase the amount of industry-sponsored research, and have National Institute of Health and private foundations target the academic health centers more (Campbell et al., 1997). Other solutions may involve specific inclusion of financial support for research and specific performance objectives/guidelines into purchase contracts between managed care organizations and hospitals.

Extensive Reporting vs. Targeted Reporting

> The concept of quality control is not new to the practice of medicine in the United States. The delivery of a high quality product is central to health care providers, hospitals, and insurers. This emphasis on quality is in part responsible for the reputation of excellence that American medicine enjoys worldwide.

Much of the current emphasis on quality stems from the movement to control rising health expenditures while maintaining the appropriate level of care. Coupled to quality is the need to ensure system efficiency. Clearly, providing unnecessary care, the waste inherent in defensive medicine, and extremes in administrative overheads served to enlarge a system that is inefficient at providing quality care at a low cost. Those involved in the provision, consumption, and purchase of health care demand that quality be cost-effective.

However, the first challenge for managed care organizations is to develop accurate assessments of quality and consumer satisfaction (Shortell and Reinhardt, 1992). The difficulty lies in the definition of quality as it is applied to certain domains in the health care field. Most would agree that when considering health care quality, the following domains need examining: access to services, how care is provided, the environment in which care is provided, outcomes of the care provided, appropriateness of care, and consumer satisfaction. Also argued is that provider satisfaction is a relevant domain in need of close assessment. Without a consensus on the definition of quality, it is extremely difficult, if not impossible, to compare various measures that do not share the same operational definitions.

In addition, it is difficult to provide any generalizations from one sample (i.e., consumers of health care plan A) to a population at large.

For numerous years, various non-related health care industries developed and used satisfaction measures. Only recently, did the need to measure consumer satisfaction reach importance in the health care field. The managed care organizations view consumer satisfaction as a vital measure of their overall performance. The difficulty with evaluating patients' perceived satisfaction is that the measurement may not accurately reflect the quality of care. Surveys and self-report scales aimed at patients tend to focus on the observable – the physical surroundings, availability of auxiliary services, the interpersonal skills of the staff, and various amenities. While these are important aspects of overall satisfaction, they tend to neglect the technical quality of the provided services. Even highly educated, health conscious patients will find it difficult to evaluate the technical quality of the health care they receive. While a patient appears highly satisfied with the cosmetic appearance of a managed care organization, that patient may actually be receiving substandard technical care. A happy patient is not always healthy, and a healthy patient is not always happy or satisfied.

The need to assess and quantify quality drove managed care organizations to closely examine how data is collected, analyzed, and utilized. The technological advancement of information systems facilitated the ease with which managed care organizations access medical care. In addition, the development of electronic medical records allowed managed care organizations to monitor utilization, develop and implement clinical pathways, and to measure various outcomes.

If measurement proves to be the key to success in the era of low cost, high quality medical care, it is necessary to examine the manner in which the data is collected. Because many managed care organizations organize on a capitation basis, records of claims tend to lack specific information concerning therapeutic interventions and outcomes. In addition, with the wide variety of managed care organizations (i.e., patient population demographics, services covered, location, provider demographics, etc.), it is virtually impossible to directly compare large data sets.

Therefore, it is important to address the issue of targeted reporting. Targeted reporting is aimed at specific data as defined by the type of measurement desired. Managed care organizations can develop and implement specific targeted reporting systems based on a defined data set. While many managed care organizations have existing data sets that are large, much of the information is administrative, not necessarily outcome or process related. Also, much of the previously collected data fails to examine variables across time and populations.

Targeted reporting has the advantage of emphasizing the development of data sets that are both reliable and valid. This becomes extremely important to the managed care organization when examining data between various providers and treatment settings. Targeted reporting also has the advantage of being able to address data collection at a specific population within the managed care organization patient base. For example, reporting can be targeted at patients with chronic illness (i.e., diabetes, congestive heart failure, chronic obstructive pulmonary disease, etc.), psychiatric illness (i.e., depression, schizophrenia, anxiety disorders, etc.), and neurological disorders (i.e., multiple sclerosis, Parkinson's, migraine headaches, etc.).

Targeted reporting also allows collection of data that is specific and usable to managed care organizations in the formulation of its marketing concept. A marketing concept resides on a market focus, customer orientation, profitability, and co-ordinated marketing. Targeted reporting can address each one of these concerns. A particular managed care organization will do best when it carefully defines its market and closely defines its consumer needs. Targeted reporting allows the managed care organization to access consumer needs from the viewpoint of the patient and thus place emphasis on what the consumer prefers and expects. In addition, since it is more costly to attract new consumers than it is to retain consumers, managed care organizations must focus on patient retention. The key to patient retention is patient satisfaction, and targeted reporting can measure satisfaction. By monitoring changing levels of patient satisfaction, the managed care organization can take earlier action and correct an actual or perceived problem. The overall concept is to use targeted reporting to measure patients' opinions, analyze and interpret the information, adjust plans, policies, or service, and plan corrective adjustment.

Targeted reporting also allows the managed care organization to evaluate efficiency control within the services it provides. By selecting specific measures including average number of patient contacts per provider per day, average time per patient contact, and number of new patient contacts per period, the managed care organization can assess the efficiency of its provider network. Managed care organizations can also select specific measures to evaluate the operational efficiency of their organization, providing insight into the cost effectiveness of the administrative infrastructure.

The challenge for managed care lies in effectively integrating its reporting systems with the need for tight quality control. As managed care organizations continue to compete for market share, it will become vitally important that all components of total quality can be effectively quantified and reported. This will demand the standardization of reporting systems not only within a particular managed care organization, but also between various managed care organizations. Targeted reporting is one solution.

Accreditation of Managed Care Organizations

accreditation

Another way to enhance the quality of a managed care organization is through **accreditation**. The National Committee for Quality Assurance (NCQA) is one independent non-profit organization dedicated to assessing and reporting on the quality of managed care plans. Another accreditation body is the Utilization Review Accreditation Commission (URAC) which focuses on the evaluation and accreditation of utilization review programs. A third non-profit accrediting body is the Joint Commission on Accreditation of Healthcare Organizations (JCAHO) which evaluates and accredits hospitals and other health care organizations. For illustrative purposes, a description of the NCQA accreditation process follows.

The NCQA's mission is to provide information that enables purchasers and consumers of managed health care to distinguish among plans based on quality, thereby allowing them to make more informed decisions. Two activities which are complementary activities for developing information to guide choices, accreditation and performance measurement, organize NCQA's efforts.

In 1996, over half of the HMOs in the U.S. applied for NCQA accreditation. NCQA gave full accreditation to 33%; 40% achieved one year accreditation; 14% received provisional accreditation; and 14% received no accreditation. The following areas are components of the NCQA Accreditation Program and a team of doctors and NCQA staff review them on site:

1. *Quality Improvement*: How well does a plan co-ordinate the various parts of its delivery system? Does the plan make sure that its members have access to health care in a reasonable

amount of time? What improvements in care and service can the plan demonstrate?

2. *Physicians Credentials*: Does the plan document the training and experience of all physicians in its network? Is a history of malpractice or fraud investigated? Are physicians' performance tracked and used for periodic evaluations?

3. *Members' Rights and Responsibilities*: Are members clearly informed about how to access health services, how to select a physician, and how to file a *complaint*?

4. *Preventive Health Services*: Does the plan support physician efforts to deliver preventive services? Are preventive tests and immunizations encouraged? Is the success of preventive care monitored?

5. *Utilization Management*: When deciding what health services are appropriate for individuals' needs, does the plan use a reasonable and consistent process? Does the plan respond to member and physician appeals when it denies payment for services? Are utilization decisions made by individuals with sufficient expertise to make them?

6. *Medical Records*: Do the medical records kept by the plan's physicians meet the standards for quality care? For example, do physicians follow-up on patients abnormal test findings?

8. *Performance*: The Health Plan Employer Data and Information Set (HEDIS) is a standardized performance measurement system that NCQA administers also.

The latest version of HEDIS, 2.5, includes general plan management information, clinical quality, access and satisfaction, membership and utilization, and plan financial performance. Areas such as medical loss ratio, immunization rates and average OB hospital stays are integral to the measurement of a plan's performance.

Currently, approximately 300 health plans are producing some HEDIS statistics and many recent 'report cards' utilize this data. An updated version is due to be finalized by the end of 1997 which will incorporate more outcome measures, acute and chronic care measures and measures that address Medicare and Medicaid.

Micromanagement vs. Macromanagement
The last 30 years saw a revolution in the control of medical management and its various outcomes. Before managed care, the medical delivery system in the United States consisted of fragmenta-

tion and increasing specialization. In addition, the United States gave little attention to efficiency and cost control. As evidenced, the medical delivery system provided care on a fee-for-service system with little regard given to overall costs. The health care system insulated providers and consumers from cost concerns, and insurance companies merely passed increasing costs to the employers.

Within this unstructured environment, the indemnity insurance companies began to attempt haphazardly to control costs through intense micromanagement. This management style was for the most part inflexible and extremely rigid. The insurance companies placed limits on professional fees, hospital fees, and procedure fees. In addition, the insurance companies set preadmission regulations and developed various guidelines concerning covered services. Physicians began to experience micromanagement of their clinical decisions. Frequently there was extensive case by case review, and challenges were made to the diagnostic database and/or the treatment plans. The insurance companies carried out this micromanagement by chart review and telephone conversations. Physicians began to feel overridden and overwhelmed by their loss of control in the clinical decision process.

Many managed care organizations observed the hostile environment created by various attempts at micromanagement and sought not to repeat a pattern that is sure to fail. Much of the change toward macromanagement is brought about by managed care organizations understanding that physicians want primary control over clinical decisions. In addition, physicians want to lessen the burden associated with the paperwork involved in billing. To this end, physicians have come to realize that the time of the individual solo practice may be over.

The philosophy of mature macromanagement can be of great benefit to the physician and the managed care organization. Prior strategies tended to focus on individual cases and restrictive utilization review in an effort to control costs. While in the short-term these practices may control spending and decrease unnecessary care, they tend to generate much hostility. In an attempt to move away from the previous model, managed care organizations are now shifting financial accountability for a patient population directly to the health care provider and the hospitals. The shift in paradigm is rooted in the concept of capitation. Capitation is an effective way to reduce waste and inefficiencies present in a health care delivery system by having the health care provider assume more of the financial risk of patient care and treatment. The challenge lies in maintaining a standard of care that is acceptable to all parties involved – the patient, the health care provider, the insurer, and the employer.

The move to macromanagement introduced the concept of management by pattern analysis. With pattern analysis there is a distinct movement away from the individual case review and challenge. Instead, there is generalized monitoring of the costs, outcomes, and processes of care in an effort to develop management based on patterns of health care delivery. While the concept of review of individual clinical decisions is the basis for micromanagement, management by patterns tends to focus review of clinical management in individual cases within the overall context of system-wide performance. System-wide performance can also be evaluated for quality of care, an important component of general satisfaction with a health care delivery system.

The movement towards macromanagement allowed greater provider autonomy – an issue at the heart of much of the hostility between providers and insurers. The mature managed care organization allows the provider to direct clinical care while assessing the care via pattern analysis. Many managed care organizations now have physician panels that deal directly with the issues of quality assurance and utilization management. In addition, there are physician panels that deal exclusively with clinical care and case management. This sharing of control and decision-making helped to increase physician satisfaction with various managed care organizations. Physician satisfaction, either directly or indirectly, most likely leads to patient satisfaction. Patient satisfaction aids the managed care organization in maintaining a strong consumer base.

Summary and Conclusions

The concept of change is one of the major challenges faced by managed care reform. Change, as a phenomenon, is inherently inconvenient, unpredictable, confusing to those involved, and most importantly, inevitable. Within the culture of organizational change, there are three major participants: the recipients of change, the agents of change, and the strategists. The strategists are typically the visionaries, the ones providing the master plan for change. The agents are the implementers, the ones providing the necessary details to bring the master plan into concrete operational focus. Finally, the recipients of change are those who are most greatly affected by the change. While to those actively seeking a power structure it may appear that the recipients are at the bottom, it must be remembered that the recipients responses are crucial to whether change is successful or not.

Change is especially problematic for managed care organizations and the medical community. Differences arise over who should be the strategist, who should be the agent and also, who should be the recipient. Still debated are the fundamental questions including, what is to be changed? in what manner? what population is affected? what are the long-term consequences? In addition, it is difficult to find one model to conceptualize the change that is taking place in health care delivery. Of the models available, Ackerman's (1986) description of transitional change, appears to most closely approximate the current trend in health care management. In transitional change, there is slow movement from a previous old state, through a transitional state, to a new state. During the transitional state, new processes and structures slowly replace current methods. Thus, during the transitional state, there are parts of both the previous state and the new evolving state.

With change necessarily comes a reaction to the change. In many cases, the reaction to significant movement from the status quo involves resistance in various forms. With the old state, there is often inertia and comfort; indeed, habits are entrenched and not easily changed. Resistance is often a reaction to actual or perceived loss of control. Finally, resistance may actually signal that an organization or system has become saturated with change and must regain a new equilibrium prior to the next series of changes.

Clearly, the challenge for managed care involves navigating the sea of change. While resistance tends to view change in a negative manner, managed care must carefully evaluate the pros and cons of each resistance movement. To dismiss resistance without a complete investigation may temporarily maintain equilibrium at the future cost of grave disequilibrium. The challenge rests in the understanding that the arrival at the new state actually signals the beginning of a new transitional state. Indeed, as the evolution of managed care continues it may become evident that certain aspects of medical delivery must always be in the transitional state to be effective and efficient for all parties involved. When activating a change solution, legitimate philosophical differences of opinions may result. Management of these differences often signals success or ushers in failure.

Glossary

Accessibility: The extent to which a member of a managed health care organization can obtain available services. For example, appointment slots may be available, but if a member cannot get through on the telephone system to schedule an appointment, the appointments are not accessible.

Accountability: Responsibility of a department or individual for achieving defined goals.

Accreditation: The formal evaluation of an organization according to accepted criteria or standards. A professional society, a non-governmental body, or a governmental agency may do accreditation. For example, NCQA accreditation is a nationally recognized evaluation that purchasers, regulators, and consumers can use to assess managed care plans.

Adverse selection: A situation in which a managed care organization enrolls a population that is disproportionally prone to higher than average utilization of benefits.

Aftercare: Individualized services following hospitalization or rehabilitation that phase the patient out of treatment in order to prevent relapse.

Agency for Health Care Policy and Research (AHCPR): An agency in the Department of Health and Human Services that is dedicated to enhancing the quality of health care on a federal level. This agency funds health care service research, conducts outcome studies and disseminates clinical practice guidelines.

Ambulatory care: Health care services that do not require hospitalization of a patient, such as those delivered at a physician's office, clinic, medical center, or outpatient facility.

American Association of Health Plans (AAHP): The Washington, D.C. based trade association that represents all managed care organizations. The association is involved in lobbying activities, educational pursuits and service to member organizations.

American Association of Preferred Provider Organizations (AAPPO): The PPOs national trade association.

Appeals mechanism: The formal process a provider of service and/or a member can use to request review of a plan decision (e.g., typically addresses benefits, utilization management, quality of care, or service issues).

Appropriateness: The extent to which a particular procedure, treatment, test, or service is clearly indicated, not excessive, adequate in quantity, and provided in the setting best suited to the needs of the patient or member.

Benchmark: For a particular indicator or performance goal, the industry measure of best performance. The benchmarking process identifies the best performance in the industry (health care or non-health care) for a particular process or outcome, determines how that performance is achieved, and applies the lessons learned to improve performance.

Beneficiary: A person designated by an insuring organization as eligible to receive insurance benefits.

Capitation: A physician is paid a fixed amount by a managed care company to care for a patient over a specific period of time. For example, a physician receives a fixed amount each month for a patient enrolled in a plan regardless of whether or not that patient is seen.

Carve-out: A decision to purchase separately a service that is typically part of an indemnity or HMO plan. For example, an HMO may 'carve-out' the behavioral health benefit and select a specialized vendor to supply these services on a stand-alone basis.

Case management: The process for identifying patients at risk for high cost care and for facilitating the development and implementation of appropriate courses of care.

Case mix: The relative frequency and intensity of hospital admissions or services reflecting different needs and uses of hospital resources. Case mix can be measured based on patients' diagnoses or the severity of their illnesses, the utilization of services, and the characteristics of the hospital.

CHAMPUS: The Civilian Health and Medical Program of the Uniformed Services provides health coverage to families of military personnel, military retirees and dependents.

Chronic: Condition or disease of long duration showing little change; opposite of acute.

Claim: Information submitted to a managed care organization by either the provider or covered person that documents medical services provided to determine the recipient of the payment.

Clinical care: The provision of health care services, including related utilization management and case management services.

Clinical outcomes: Outcome data on clinical services and procedures often dependent upon targeted goals and objective measurements.

Clinical privileges: Authorization by the governing body for an individual to provide specific patient care and treatment services in the organization (within well-defined limits), based on the individual's expertise, education, training, experience, and competence.

Comorbidity: Co-existing (usually chronic) conditions that may affect overall health and functional status beyond the effect(s) of the condition under consideration.

Complaint: Expression of dissatisfaction by a member. Generally, complaints are oral expressions of dissatisfaction and grievances are written expressions of dissatisfaction.

Concurrent review: Assessment of the need for continued inpatient care for hospitalized patients.

COBRA: The Consolidated Omnibus Budget Reconciliation Act requires employers to offer the opportunity to purchase continuation of health care coverage under the companies medical plan to terminated employees.

Communitywide program: A type of prevention program in which all of the people in a given geographic area receive the preventive intervention.

Continuity of clinical care: The provision of care by the same set of clinicians to a member over time or, if the same providers are not available over time, a mechanism to provide appropriate clinical information in a timely fashion to the clinicians who continue to provide the same type and level of care.

Co-ordination of clinical care: The mechanisms assuring that the member and clinicians have access to, and take into consideration, all the required information on the member's conditions and treatments to assure that he or she receives appropriate health care services.

Co-payment: The out-of-pocket fixed expense (e.g., $10) that a member must pay to a managed care organization at the time that health care is rendered.

Credentialing: The process by which the managed care organization authorizes, contracts with, or employs clinicians who are licensed to practice independently, to provide services to its members. Eligibility is determined by the extent to which applicants meet defined requirements for education, licensure, professional standing, service availability and accessibility, and conformance with managed care organization utilization and quality management requirements.

Criteria: Systematically developed statements used to assess the appropriateness of specific health care decisions, services, and outcomes.

Customer service: The administrative systems that enroll the member, provide information about how to utilize the managed care organization, handle member concerns, and assist the member in receiving clinical services.

Customary, prevailing and reasonable charges: A Medicare reimbursement method which pays physicians according to the following criteria: a physician's median charge in a recent time period, a physician's actual charge or the 75th percentile of charges in a recent time period.

Day treatment center: A behavioral health care setting that provides an interdisciplinary program of medical and therapeutic services at least three hours per day, five days per week. Day treatment centers may be either freestanding or part of a broader behavioral health care or medical system.

Deductible: In a given period of time, the initial amount that a consumer must pay for medical services before the third party payer is responsible for the remaining amount.

Delegation: A formal process by which a managed care organization gives a contractor the authority to perform certain functions on its behalf, such as credentialing, utilization management, and quality improvement. Although a managed care organization can delegate the authority to perform a function, it cannot delegate the responsibility for assuring the function is performed appropriately.

Diagnostic and Statistical Manual – 4th edition: American Psychiatric Association's manual of diagnostic criteria and terminology, widely accepted as the common language of mental health clinicians and researchers.

Diagnosis-Related Groups (DRGs): A system of classifying an inpatient stay into groups for purposes of payment under the medicare system.

Discharge planning: The process of developing a care regimen for a patient leaving institutional clinical care, including appropriate timing and follow-up examinations and treatment.

Disease state management: An approach to health care that utilizes disease-specific practice guidelines that are built into computer models that practitioners can use to assist them in patient treatment planning.

Dual diagnosis: Co-existence of more than one disorder in an individual patient. Commonly refers to a patient who is diagnosed with mental illness in conjunction with substance abuse.

Employee Assistance Program: A program that a corporation provides to its employees to assist them with mental health or substance abuse issues.

Employer mandate: A requirement established by state or federal standards that employers with more than 25 employees who provide health insurance must offer an HMO plan as an alternative.

Epidemiology: A subspecialty within public health concerned with determining who becomes ill, how many people have a given illness, why people become ill and what can be done to stop them from becoming ill.

ERISA: The Employee Retirement Income Security Act, allows among several provisions, a self-funded plan to avoid paying premium taxes or otherwise comply with state laws and regulations concerning insurance.

Evidence based medicine: Physicians are trained to search databases for sound medical research to determine tests and treatments that have been evaluated with randomized controlled trials.

Exclusive Provider Organization (EPO): An EPO combines the features of HMOs and PPOs but requires that members remain inside the network to receive benefits.

Fee-for-service: The traditional way physicians have been paid for services with an established fee for each service provided, also referred to as an indemnity health plan.

Formulary: A catalog of the pharmaceutical approved for use in an organization; a list of the names of the drugs and information regarding dosage, contra-indications, and unit dispensing size.

Gatekeeper model: A situation in which a 'gatekeeper' (e.g., a primary care physician), serves as the patient's initial contact for medical care and referrals.

Governing body: The individuals, group, or agency with ultimate authority and responsibility for the overall operation of the organization.

Grievance: A written expression of member dissatisfaction.

Group Model HMO: An HMO that provides health care services by contracting with a medical group.

Guardianship: The legal appointment of a responsible person (guardian) who controls or manages the affairs of an individual who is incapable of exercising rational judgment or giving informed consent. Guardianship arrangements may apply to the care and treatment of mentally ill, mentally retarded, or minor patients.

Health Maintenance Organization (HMO): An entity that provides, offers or arranges for coverage of designated health services needed by plan members for a fixed, prepaid premium. There are four basic models of HMOs: group model, individual practice association, network model, and staff model.

Health promotion: Its focus is on the enhancement of well-being rather than illness and can be provided to individuals, groups or even larger populations.

Health protection: A public health mechanism that seeks to reduce the number of health hazards in the environment through the use of public regulatory activities.

High-risk program: A type of prevention program that focuses on high-risk populations, rather than events. An example would be children of alcoholics.

ICD-9-CM (International Classification of Diseases, 9th revision): The classification of disease by diagnosis and coded into six digit numbers.

Important aspects of care: Clinical or customer service activities that involve a high volume of patients, that entail a high degree of risk for patients, and/or that tend to produce problems for patients or staff. Such activities are deemed most important for purposes of ongoing monitoring and evaluation.

Indemnity health insurance plan: Traditional health care insurance that reimburses the patient for procedural services they have paid. For example, Blue Cross/Blue Shield is an example of this type of plan.

Independent Practice Association (IPA): An HMO that contracts with individual physicians or with independent associations of physicians that have been formed for the purpose of providing services to managed health care organizations.

Indicator: A defined, measurable variable used to monitor the quality or appropriateness of an important aspect of patient care. Indicators can be activities, events, occurrences, or outcomes for which data can be collected to allow comparison with a threshold, a benchmark, or prior performance. Clinical indicators are of two types: outcome indicators and process indicators.

Institutional settings: Any setting in which the patient spends five or more hours per day. This includes acute care facilities, skilled nursing facilities, residential treatment programs, and day treatment programs.

Integrated health care system: A system of health care providers that combines independent managed care services into a seamless delivery system. Components could include employee assistance services, a telephone counseling triage, utilization management, behavioral treatment networks, claims payment, and data management.

Licensed independent practitioner: Any individual permitted by law and by the organization to provide individual/patient care services without direction or supervision, within the scope of the individual's licensure or certification, and in accordance with individually granted clinical privileges.

Managed health care: A system of health care delivery that attempts to manage the cost and quality of health care as well as access to that care.

Managed Behavioral Healthcare Organization (MBHCO): A system of health care delivery that influences utilization and cost of services and measures performance in the areas of mental and/or psychoactive substance abuse disorders. The goal is a system that delivers value by giving people access to quality, cost-effective healt care.

Medical management systems: Systems designed to assure that members receive appropriate clinical services. Medical management systems include, but are not limited to, utilization management, quality improvement, case management, and complaint and grievance resolution.

Medical record: The record in which clinical information related to the provision of physical, social, and mental health services is recorded and stored.

Medicaid: A program to provide health insurance for people who live in poverty administered by the state government. Both the federal and state government provides funding. There are no premiums.

Medicare: A program that provides health insurance for people age 65 years and older and some younger disabled individuals. Medicare has two parts: A which pays for hospital care and B which pays for physician care. Part A does not charge a premium but Part B does. There are also deductibles for hospital care as well as restrictions.

Members: Individuals for whom the managed care organization has a contractual obligation to provide, or arrange for the, provision of health services.

Milestone program: A type of prevention program where every individual in a population who reaches a certain hurdle is a member of the target group. An example would be becoming a parent for the first time, or getting fired.

Mixed Model HMO: A combination of the IPA Model, the Group Model, the Network Model or the Staff Model. Different models are merged under a larger umbrella organization.

Multidisciplinary: Determination of treatment plans and delivery of care through professionals with a wide range of specialties.

National Practitioner Data Bank (NPDB): Located at P.O. Box 6048, Camarillo, CA 93011-6048, this data bank is the repository of information about settled or lost malpractice suits and adverse acts, sanctions, or restrictions against the practice privileges of a physician.

Network Model HMO: A health plan that contracts with multiple practitioner groups to deliver health care to its members.

Open enrollment period: A period, which usually occurs once a year, when an employee may change health plans.

Oversight: The monitoring and direction of a set of activities by individuals responsible for the execution of the activities, resulting in the achievement of desired outcomes.

Over-utilization: Provision of services that were not clearly indicated, or provision of services that were indicated in either excessive amounts or in a higher-level setting than required.

Partial-hospitalization program: A program that provides services to persons who spend only part of a 24-hour period in the facility. Partial-hospitalization programs do not provide overnight care.

Peer review: Evaluation or review of the performance of colleagues by professionals with similar types and degrees of expertise (e.g., the evaluation of one physician's practice by another physician). The term is used for both utilization management and quality assurance activities.

Performance goals: The desired level of achievement of standards of care or service. These may be expressed as desired minimum performance levels (thresholds), industry best performance benchmarks), or the permitted variance from the standard. Performance goals usually are not static but change as performance improves and/or the standard of care is refined.

Performance measure: A specific measure of how well a health plan does in providing health services to its enrolled population. Can be used as a measure of quality.

Physician Hospital Organization (PHO): An organization of hospitals and their attending medical staff that have joined together to contract with managed care plans.

Point-of-service: A plan which permits members to go outside of the plan for services at an additional charge.

Population-based strategies: Analyses which measure compliance to a quality indicator across all at-risk members in the managed care organization. For example, a population-based pediatric immunization study includes all at-risk children in the denominator of the compliance rate, not only those who have accessed a health delivery site.

Practice guidelines: Systematically developed statements to assist practitioner and patient decisions about appropriate health care for specific clinical circumstances. Practice guidelines are usually based on such authoritative sources as clinical literature and expert consensus.

Preferred Provider Organization (PPO): A partnership between a hospital and a group of health care professionals to provide services to a patient pool. PPOs represent a combination of the traditional indemnity and HMO models.

Prevention: An approach to disease management which emphasizes a reduction in the number of people who already have a disorder, or which emphasizes reductions in the number of people who develop the disorder anew.

Primary care physician: General practice physician, family physician, general internist or pediatrician who is responsible for providing and co-ordinating all the member's health care services. This person authorizes all referrals to specialists and payment is contingent upon this authorization.

Prior review/authorization/certification/determination: Prior assessment that proposed services, such as hospitalization, are appropriate for a particular patient. Payment for services also depends on whether the patient and the category of service are covered by the member's benefit plan.

Providers: Individuals licensed, certified or authorized by law to render professional health services directly to members. For example, physicians, physicians' assistants, nurse practitioners, chiropractors, and dentists are included in the term.

Quality assessment: Measurement and evaluation of the quality of medical care for individuals, groups, or populations.

Quality improvement: The effort to improve the level of performance of a key process within an organization which is often annually updated. Opportunities to improve care and service are found primarily by examining the systems and processes by which care and services are provided.

Quality of Care: The degree to which health services for individuals and populations increase the likelihood of desired health outcomes and are consistent with current professional knowledge.

Recidivism: The frequency that a patient with the same presenting problem returns for inpatient hospital treatment.

Referral: The sending of an individual (1) from one clinician to another clinician or specialist, (2) from one setting or service to another, (3) by one physician (the referring physician) to another physician(s) (or some other resource) either for consultation or care.

Report cards: A mechanism utilized by the managed care industry to evaluate the performance of various health plans. Also, they are sometimes used to evaluate a physician performance of his/her adherence to a managed care plan's policy.

Retrospective review: Assessment of the appropriateness of medical services on a case-by-case or aggregate basis after the services have been provided.

Risk analysis: The evaluation of expected health care costs for a prospective group in order to determine the most appropriate benefit level, product and price that a carrier should offer.

Risk pool: Funds withheld from a providers' fees (usually 20%) to cover budget overruns and to increase sensitivity to cost pressures.

Sanction: A reprimand of a participating provider for some aspect of health care delivery.

Staff Model HMO: An HMO that employs health care providers on a salary basis and sees members in its own medical facilities for the most part.

Standards: Authoritative statements of (1) minimum levels of acceptable performance or results, (2) excellent level of performance or results, or (3) the range of acceptable performance or results.

Telemedicine: A system that electronically transports a consulting physician's expertise to a site at a distant facility where it is needed. The most common clinical uses are diagnostic consults, data transmissions and management of chronic illnesses.

Third party payer: A private or public organization such as a commercial insurer that pays for healthcare expenses of another entity.

Threshold for Evaluation: The base or minimum acceptable level of performance; often perceived as a starting point.

Treatment plan: A written action plan, based on assessment data, that identifies the individual's/patient's clinical needs, the strategy for providing services to meet those needs, treatment goals and objectives, and the criteria for terminating the specified interventions.

Triage: A military term which is used to classify the sick or injured according to severity in order to ensure the most efficient use of medical resources.

Underutilization: Failure to provide appropriate and/or indicated services, or provision of an inadequate quantity or lower level of services than required (see appropriateness).

Usual, Customary and Reasonable Fee (UCR): Fees judged to be the 'going rate' for a particular service in a specific geographical area.

Utilization management: Evaluation and determination of the appropriateness of patient use of medical care resources, and provision of any needed assistance to clinician and/or member, to ensure appropriate use of resources. Includes prior authorization, concurrent review, retrospective review, discharge planning, and case management.

References

Ackermann, L. D. 1986. Optimizing identity: A marketing imperative for health care management. Journal of Health Care Marketing. 6 Jun 2: 49–56.

Adelson, A. 1997. Health Plans With Choice: Good Deals? New York Times. Business Section, p. 15.

American Nurses Association, June, 1997. Proceedings of the house of delegates forum on managed care. Washington, D.C.

American Political Network, February, 1997. Kiddiecare: Will The Clinton Plan Take Off? Alexandria, VA: National Journal Company.

Blendon, R. J. and Hyams, T. S., eds. 1992. Reforming the system: Containing health care costs in an era of universal coverage. The future of American health care. Volume II. Washington, D.C.: Faulkner and Gray's Healthcare Information Center.

Bloom, B. 1985. Community mental health: A general introduction. Second edition. Monterey, CA: Brooks/Cole.

Bodenheimer, T. and Grumbach, K. 1995. The reconfiguration of U.S. medicine. Journal of the American Medical Association. 274: 85–89.

Bodenheimer, T. 1997. The Oregon Health Plan – Lessons for the Nation (Second of two parts) The New England Journal of Medicine. 337: 720–723.

Bok, D. 1996. The state of the nation. Cambridge, Massachusetts: Harvard University Press.

Boland, P., ed. 1992. Making managed healthcare work: A practical guide to strategies and solutions. Gaithersburg, MD: Aspen Publishers.

Bordley, J. and Harvey, A. 1976. Two centuries of American medicine. Philadelphia: W. B. Saunders.

Burton, W. and Hoy, D. 1993. First Chicago's integrated health data management computer system. Managed Care Quarterly. 1: 18–23.

Campbell, E., Weissman, J. and Blumenthal, D. 1997. Relationship between market competition and the activities and attitudes of medical school faculty. Journal of the American Medical Association. 278: 222–226.

Caplan, G. 1964. Principles of preventive psychiatry. New York: Basic Books.

Cassell, E. J. 1997. Doctoring: The nature of primary care medicine. London: Oxford University Press.

Centers for Disease Control. 1996. Morbidity and mortality weekly report. Washington, D.C.: Government Printing Office.

Charap, M. 1981. The periodic health examination: genesis of a myth. Annals of Internal Medicine. 95: 733–735.

Clinton, W. J. 1998. *The state of the union address.* 27 January, Washington, D.C.: The White House.

Cooper, R. 1994. Seeking a balanced physician workforce for the 21st century. Journal of the American Medical Association. 272: 680–687.

Corcoran, K. and Vandiver, V. 1996. Maneuvering the maze of managed care: Skills for mental health practitioners. New York: The Free Press.

Dellinger, Anne M., ed. 1992. Health Care facilities law. Critical issues for hospitals, HMOs and extended care facilities. Boston, MA: Little, Brown and Company.

Dohrenwend, B., Dohrenwend, B. S., Gould, M., Link, B., Neugebauer, R. and Wunschhititzig, R. 1979. Mental illness in the United States. New York: Praeger.

Field, M. and Shapiro, H. 1995. Employment and health benefits: A connection at risk. Washington, D.C.: National Academy Press.

Finocchio, L., Bailiff, P., Grant, R. and O'Neil, E. 1995. Professional competencies in the changing health care system: Physicians' views on the importance and adequacy of formal training in medical school. Academic Medicine, 70: 1023–1028.

Flexner, A. 1972. Medical education in the United States and Canada: A report to the Carnegie foundation for the advancement of teaching. New York: Arno Press. [c1910].

Freudenheim, M. 1995. An exam for home health care. The New York Times, 15 September, sec. D, p. 1–2.

Freudenheim, M. 1997. Health care providers say companies gain from float. The New York Times, 17 April, sec. C, p. 1.

Freudenheim, M. 1998. Study shows dominance of managed care plans in '97. The New York Times, 20 January, sec. D, p. 8.

Fulton, J. 1993. Canada's health system: Bordering on the possible. Washington, D.C.: Faulkner and Gray.

Goldstein, A. 1998. Florida curbs HMOs powers. The Washington Post, 24 June, sec. A, p. 1 and p. 6.

Goodman, J. C. and Musgrave, G. L. 1994. Patient power: Solving America's health care crisis. Washington, D.C.: Cato Institute.

Gold, M. 1995. HMO organizations: Critical issues raised by restructuring delivery for health systems reform. In Managed Care: The Journal of Ambulatory Care Management, edited by S. B. Goldsmith. Gaithersburg, MD: Aspen Publishers.

Goodman, M., Brown, J. and Deitz, P. 1992. Managing managed care. A mental health practitioners survival guide. Washington, D.C.: American Psychiatric Press.

Graig, L. A. 1993. Health of nations: An international perspective on U.S. health care reform. Second edn. Washington, D.C.: Congressional Quarterly Inc.

Griffith, J. R. 1995. The well managed health care organization. Ann Arbor, MI: Health Administration Press.

Hardy, A. M., Rauch, K., Echenberg, D., Morgan, W. and Curran, J. 1986. The economic impact of the first 10,000 cases of acquired immunodeficiency syndrome in the U.S. Journal of the American Medical Association. 255: 209–211.

Hellinger, F. 1993. The lifetime cost of treating a person with HIV. Journal of the American Medical Association. 270: 474–478.

Henig, R. M. 1997. The People's Health. Washington, D.C.: Joseph Henry Press.

Himmelstein, D. and Woolhandler, S. 1994. The national health program book. Monroe, ME: Common Courage Press.

Hobbs, N. 1975. The futures of children. San Francisco: Jossey-Bass.

Hough, R., Gongla, P., Brown, V. and Goldston, S. 1985. Psychiatric epidemiology and prevention. Los Angeles: University of California, Neuropsychiatric Institute.

Huefner, R. P. and Battin, M. P., Eds. 1992. Changing to national health care. Salt Lake City: University of Utah Press.

Hurley, R. E., Freund, D. A. and Paul, J. E. 1993. Managed care in Medicaid. Lessons for policy and program design. Ann Arbor, MI: Health Administration Press.

Iglehart, J. 1993. The American health care system: Community hospitals. New England Journal of Medicine. 329: 372–376.

Institute of Medicine. 1996. Telemedicine. Washington, D.C.: National Academy Press.

Institute of Medicine. 1996. 2020 Vision: Health in the 21st century. Washington, DC: National Academy Press.

James, G. 1997. Making managed care work: Strategies for local market dominance. Chicago, IL: Irwin Professional Publishing.

Kelch, B. P., Amos, W. L. Jr. and Elden, D. L. 1992. The PPO evaluation manual. Reston, VA: American Accreditation Program/MedStrategies, Inc.

Kongstvedt, P. R., ed. 1997. Chapter 8 in The essentials of managed health care. Second edn. Gaithersburg, MD: Aspen Publishers.

Marmor, T. R. 1994. Understanding health reform. New Haven, Connecticut: Yale University Press.

Masi, D. and Caplan, R. 1992. Employee assistance programs. In Managed mental health care. Administrative and clinical issues. Edited by Feldman, J. and Fitzpatrick, R., Washington, D.C.: American Psychiatric Press.

Meyer, G. S. and Blumenthal, D. 1996. TennCare and academic medical centers. Journal of the American Medical Association. 276: 672–676.

Miller, R. and Luft, H. 1994. Managed care plan performance since 1980: A literature analysis. Journal of the American Medical Association. 271: 1512–1519.

Moore, G. T., Inui, T. S., Ludden, J. M. and Schoembaum, S. C. 1994. The teaching HMO: A new academic partner. Academic Medicine. 69: 595–600.

Morreim, E. 1997. Managed care, ethics, and academic health centers: Maximizing potential, minimizing drawbacks. Academic Medicine 72: 332–338.

Moy, E., Mazzaschi, A., Levin, R., Blake, D. and Griner, P. 1997. Relationship between National Institutes of Health research awards to U.S. medical schools and managed care market penetration. Journal of the American Medical Association. 278: 217–221.

Mrazek, P. and Haggerty, R., eds. 1994. Reducing risks for mental disorders: Frontiers for preventive intervention research. Washington D.C.: National Academy Press.

National Committee for Quality Assurance. 1993. Health plan data and information set 2.0. Washington, D.C.: NCQA.

National Committee for Quality Assurance. 1995. Hedis 2.5 updated specifications for hedis 2.0. Washington, D.C.: NCQA

National Committee for Quality Assurance. 1995. Standards for accreditation. Washington, D.C.: NCQA.

Pauly, M. V., Eisenberg, J. M., Radany, M. H. 1992. Paying physicians: options for controlling cost, volume, and intensity of services. Ann Arbor, MI: Health Administration Press.

Pew Health Professions Commission, 1995. Health professions education and managed care: Challenges and necessary responses. Report of the Advisory Panel on Health Professions Education and Managed Care.

Raffel, M. W. and Raffel, N. K. 1994. The U.S. health system: Origins and functions fourth edn. Albany, NY: Delmar.

Rickel, A. U. and Becker, E. 1998. Keeping children from harm's way. Washington, D.C.: American Psychological Association.

Rovner, J. 1997. Managed care and medicare: How to make them work for you. Modern Maturity Magazine. 40: 35–80.

Rubin, J. 1992. Mental health care and substance abuse: A review on insurance coverage and utilization. Upland, PA: Diane Publishing Co.

Ruskin, A. 1997. Capitation: The legal implications of using capitation to affect physician decision-making processes. Journal of Contemporary Health Law and Policy. 13: 391–421.

Sabin, J. E. 1996. Is managed care ethical care? In Lazarus, A. (ed.), Controversies in managed mental health care. Washington, D.C.: American Psychiatric Press.

Shenkin, B. 1995. The independent practice association in theory and practice. Journal of the American Medical Association 273: 1937–1942.

Shortell, S. M. and Reinhardt, U. E., eds. 1992. Improving health policy and management: Nine critical research issues for the 1990s. Ann Arbor, MI: Health Administration Press.

Smilie, J. G. 1991. Can physicians manage the quality and costs of health care: The story of the Permanente Medical Group. NY: McGraw-Hill, Inc.

Starr, P. 1992. The logic of health care reform, transforming American medicine for the better. Knoxville, TN: Grand Rounds Press/Whittle Direct Books.

Stevens, D. P., Leach, D. C., Warden, G. L. and Cherniack, N. S. 1996. A strategy for coping with change: An affiliation between a medical school and a managed care health system. Academic Medicine 71: 133–137.

The Pepper Commission. 1990. Call for Action: Final Report. Washington, D.C.: Government Printing Office.

Todd, W. E. and Nash, D. 1997. Disease management: A systems approach to improving patient outcomes. Chicago, IL: American Hospital Publishing Inc.

Traska, Maria. 1992. Health care and the electronic superhighway: A provider perspective on electronic data interchange and automated medical payment, Faulkner & Gray research report 92–3. Washington, D. C.: Faulkner & Gray.

U.S. Bureau of the Census, Last Revision: May 13, 1997.

U.S. Department of Commerce. 1976. Historical statistics of the United States Part 1. Washington, D.C.: Government Printing Office.

U.S. Department of Commerce. 1996. Statistical abstract of the United States 1996. Washington, D.C.: Government Printing Office.

U.S. Department of Health and Human Services. 1995. Health care financing review, Fall, 1995. Washington, D.C.: Government Printing Office.

U.S. Department of Health and Human Services. 1997. Health United States 1996–97. Washington, DC: Government Printing Office.

U.S. Senate Special Committee on Aging. 1989. Long-term care in rural America: a family and health policy challenge, part 6. Washington, D.C.: Government Printing Office.

U.S. Senate Select Committee on Aging. 1991. *Aging America: Trends and projections.* Washington, D.C.: Government Printing Office.

Veloski, M., Barzansky, B., Nash, D., Bastacky, S. and Stevens, D. 1996. Medical student education in managed care settings. Journal of the American Medical Association. 276: 667–671.

Vogel, David E. 1992. Family physicians and managed care: A view to the 90s. Kansas City, MO: American Academy of Family Physicians.

Washington Outlook. 1993. AIDS tab to grow. Hospitals 67: 8.

Weiner, J. 1994. Financing long-term care. Journal of the American Medical Association 271: 1525–1529.

Zelman, W. A. 1996. The changing health care marketplace. San Francisco, California: Jossey-Bass, Inc.

Zuger, A. 1997. New way of doctoring: By the book. New York Times, 16 December, sec. C, p. 1 and 7.

Subject Index

Group model, overview 36, 101
Guardianship, definition 101

Health insurance
 case study of managed care options 50, 51
 fee-for-service providers 33, 100
 history 10, 11
 indemnity plan 33, 102
 micromanagement in cost control 91, 92
Health Insurance Portability and Accountability Act of 1996 28
Health maintenance organization (HMO)
 case study
  asthma attack 64–66
  back problems 67–69
  breast cancer 66, 67
  managed care option selection 50, 51
 cost control 35, 53
 definition 101
 enrollment trends 35, 79
 gatekeeper model 34, 84, 100
 group model 36, 101
 independent practice association 36
 members 34
 mixed model 37, 38
 network model 36, 37, 104
 primary care physician 34
 specialty systems
  mental health 41, 42
  pharmacy benefits 42, 43
 staff model 37, 107
Health Maintenance Organization Act of 1973 11
Health Plan Employer Data and Information Set (HEDIS) 91
Health Professions Education Assistance Act of 1963 4
Health promotion 75, 101
Health protection 75, 101
Health Security Bill 28
HEDIS, see Health Plan Employer Data and Information Set
High-risk program, disease prevention 76, 101
Hill Burton Act of 1946 7, 8
History, managed care
 disease pattern changes 20–22
 driving forces for development 17, 18

expenditures 22–27
financing Medicare and Medicaid 11–15
Health Maintenance Organization Act of 1973 11
health insurance 10, 11
hospitals 5–10
medical education 3–5
overview 1–3, 15, 16
HMO, see Health maintenance organization
Hospital, see also Academic medical center
 expenditures on services 25, 32
 history
  academic health centers 8, 9
  antiseptic surgery 5
  community hospitals 9, 10
  depression era 7
  diagnostics 6
  Hill Burton Act of 1946 7, 8
  peer review 6, 7, 104
  technology in medical practice 5
  trends in numbers 8
  types of hospitals 6
 mergers 54, 55
 partial hospitalization 54, 104

IHS, see Integrated healthcare system
Indemnity plan, see Health insurance
Independent practice association (IPA), overview 36
Indicator, definition 102
Institutional setting, definition 102
Integrated healthcare system (IHS), overview 40, 41, 102
IPA, see Independent practice association

JCAHO, see Joint Commission on Accreditation of Healthcare Organizations
Japan, health care system 31, 32
Joint Commission on Accreditation of Healthcare Organizations (JCAHO) 90

Licensed independent practioner, definition 102
Long-term care, expenditures 26, 27

Macromanagement, cost control 92, 93
Managed behavioral health care organizations 41, 102, 103

high-risk program 76
milestone program 75
tertiary prevention 72, 73
Prior authorization
case management 55, 56
drug treatments 43
Prior review, definition 105
Provider, definition 105

Quality management
accountability 59, 60, 95
assessment 106
audits 61
clinical outcomes 60, 97
consumer rights legislation 60, 61
improvement 106
oversight 60
performance measurement 60
reporting, extensive versus targeted 87–90

Recidivism, definition 106
Referral, definition 106
Report card, functions 58, 106
Retrospective review 56, 106
Risk factors
modifiable risk factors 77
precipitating risk factors 77, 78
predisposing risk factors 77

unmodifiable risk factors 77
Risk pool, definition 106

Sanction, definition 106
Staff model, overview 37, 107
States
health care reform programs 29
legislation of managed care 82, 83

Targeted reporting, advantages 88–90
Telemedicine 63, 107
Third party payor, definition 107
Threshold for evaluation, definition 107
Treatment planning 55, 107
Triage, patients 55, 107

UCR fee, see Usual customary and reasonable fee
Underutilization, definition 107
United Kingdom, health care system 30, 31
Unmodifiable risk factors 77
Usual customary and reasonable (UCR) fee
definition 107
preferred provider organizations 39
setting 34
Utilization management 55, 107
Utilization Review Accreditation Commission (URAC), accreditation 90